Homework Success
for Children with ADHD

THE GUILFORD SCHOOL PRACTITIONER SERIES

Editors

Stephen N. Elliott, PhD, *University of Wisconsin–Madison*
Joseph C. Witt, PhD, *Louisiana State University, Baton Rouge*

Recent Volumes

HOMEWORK SUCCESS FOR CHILDREN WITH ADHD:
A FAMILY–SCHOOL INTERVENTION PROGRAM
  Thomas J. Power, James L. Karustis, and Dina F. Habboushe

CONDUCTING SCHOOL-BASED ASSESSMENTS OF CHILD AND ADOLESCENT BEHAVIOR
  Edward S. Shapiro and Thomas R. Kratochwill, Editors

DESIGNING PRESCHOOL INTERVENTIONS: A PRACTITIONER'S GUIDE
  David W. Barnett, Susan H. Bell, and Karen T. Carey

EFFECTIVE SCHOOL INTERVENTIONS
  Natalie Rathvon

DSM-IV DIAGNOSIS IN THE SCHOOLS
  Alvin E. House

MEDICATIONS FOR SCHOOL-AGE CHILDREN: EFFECTS ON LEARNING AND BEHAVIOR
  Ronald T. Brown and Michael G. Sawyer

ADVANCED APPLICATIONS OF CURRICULUM-BASED MEASUREMENT
  Mark R. Shinn, Editor

BRIEF INTERVENTION FOR SCHOOL PROBLEMS:
COLLABORATING FOR PRACTICAL SOLUTIONS
  John J. Murphy and Barry L. Duncan

ACADEMIC SKILLS PROBLEMS: DIRECT ASSESSMENT AND INTERVENTION,
SECOND EDITION
  Edward S. Shapiro

SOCIAL PROBLEM SOLVING: INTERVENTIONS IN THE SCHOOLS
  Maurice J. Elias and Steven E. Tobias

INSTRUCTIONAL CONSULTATION TEAMS: COLLABORATING FOR CHANGE
  Sylvia A. Rosenfield and Todd A. Gravois

ENTRY STRATEGIES FOR SCHOOL CONSULTATION
  Edward S. Marks

SCHOOL INTERVENTIONS FOR CHILDREN OF ALCOHOLICS
  Bonnie K. Nastasi and Denise M. DeZolt

ADHD IN THE SCHOOLS: ASSESSMENT AND INTERVENTION STRATEGIES
  George J. DuPaul and Gary Stoner

Homework Success for Children with ADHD

A FAMILY–SCHOOL INTERVENTION PROGRAM

Thomas J. Power
James L. Karustis
Dina F. Habboushe

Foreword by Susan M. Sheridan

THE GUILFORD PRESS
New York   London

© 2001 The Guilford Press
A Division of Guilford Publications, Inc.
72 Spring Street, New York, NY 10012
www.guilford.com

Printed in the United States of America

This book is printed on acid-free paper.

Last digit is print number: 9 8 7 6 5 4 3 2 1

Library of Congress Cataloging-in-Publication Data

Power, Thomas J.
    Homework success for children with ADHD / Thomas J. Power, James L. Karustis,
Dina F. Habboushe ; foreword by Susan M. Sheridan.
        p. cm.—(The Guilford school practitioner series)
    Includes bibliographical references (p.) and index.
    ISBN 1-57230-616-5 (pbk.)
    1. Attention-deficit-disordered children—Education. 2. Attention-deficit
hyperactivity disorder. 3. Homework. 4. Home and school. I. Karustis, James L.
II. Habboushe, Dina F. III. Title. IV. Series.

LC4713.2 .P69 2001
371.93—dc21
                                                                    00-51383

*To our parents, spouses, and children for the love
that energized and inspired us throughout this project*

*To our colleagues in the Center for Management of ADHD
at The Children's Hospital of Philadelphia for their
friendship, creativity, and commitment to children and families*

*And to the families who have participated in the Homework
Success Program for teaching us to be hopeful amidst the
challenges of coping with ADHD*

About the Authors

Thomas J. Power, PhD, Associate Professor of School Psychology in Pediatrics at the University of Pennsylvania School of Medicine, is Director of the Center for Management of ADHD at The Children's Hospital of Philadelphia. Dr. Power is Associate Editor of *School Psychology Review* and author of numerous journal articles and book chapters pertaining to ADHD. He is coauthor of the *ADHD Rating Scale–IV: Checklists, Norms, and Clinical Interpretation* and *The Clinician's Practical Guide to Attention-Deficit/Hyperactivity Disorder.* Dr. Power has spent many years providing services to children with ADHD and helping his three children with their homework.

James L. Karustis, PhD, is a licensed psychologist and nationally certified school psychologist in private practice in southeastern Pennsylvania. He was formerly a psychologist at Children's Seashore House of The Children's Hospital of Philadelphia and a Clinical Associate in Pediatrics at the University of Pennsylvania School of Medicine. Dr. Karustis is a well-known speaker and writer on ADHD in the Delaware Valley and is currently an officer with both the Pennsylvania Psychological Association and the Association of School Psychologists of Pennsylvania. Dr. Karustis is a devoted father and frequent traveler to India. He can be reached through his website at *http://www.karustis.com.*

Dina F. Habboushe, PhD, Post-Doctoral Fellow in Pediatric Psychology at The Children's Hospital of Philadelphia, conducted her doctoral studies at MCP Hahnemann University in Philadelphia and served her internship at Harvard Medical School/Children's Hospital in Boston. Dr. Habboushe's clinical and research interests include behavioral interventions for children and families coping with ADHD and related problems. She also specializes in the promotion of adherence and coping strategies for children with chronic illnesses and disorders.

About the Contributors

Tracy E. Costigan, PhD, Training Department, SPSS Inc., Washington, DC

Sheeba Daniel-Crotty, PhD, Department of Child and Adolescent Psychiatry, University of Chicago, Chicago, Illinois

Suzanne G. Goldstein, MA, Department of Clinical and Health Psychology, MCP Hahnemann University, Philadelphia, Pennsylvania

Stephen S. Leff, PhD, Department of Psychology, The Children's Hospital of Philadelphia, Philadelphia, Pennsylvania

Foreword

Homework. Children with attention–deficit/hyperactivity disorder (ADHD). Therein lies a challenging combination. As Power, Karustis, and Habboushe so aptly note, several commercial programs are available to help children with homework problems. Likewise, several interventions are known to be effective for children with ADHD. To date, though, no source has been available that presents homework strategies that are effective for the unique characteristics of children who have attentional problems. This book offers that and much more.

I have long believed that, to be a seminal resource on a topic, a work must attend to important theoretical underpinnings, practical considerations, and empirical referents. Psychologists have a professional and ethical responsibility when working with children, families, and schools to ensure that their models of service are grounded in all of these. That is, any model devoid of solid conceptual, practical, or empirical bases is not likely to benefit the field of psychology and the constituencies it serves. The Homework Success Program, articulated clearly in this carefully crafted resource, advances this principle explicitly.

THEORETICAL PERSPECTIVES

I am a systems thinker. It is hard for me to consider working with a child or family exclusive of the multiple settings and systems within which the individual child or family unit functions. The Homework Success Program is grounded in a multisystemic, ecological approach that recognizes the importance of the interconnectedness among systems in a child's life (Bronfenbrenner, 1977). All key players have a role in the program: parents, teachers, medical professionals, and psychologists. When it comes to homework, parents and teachers are perhaps the most important adults in a child's daily life, being responsible for the development of effective homework and implementation of the program at home. Medical professionals and psychologists in schools and agencies support children with ADHD and thus are also instrumental in their success. The

Homework Success Program effectively merges these significant individuals in a comprehensive, coordinated manner. The notion of parents and teachers working collaboratively and with the support of doctors and psychologists to address academic and homework concerns simply makes good sense.

PRACTICE PERSPECTIVES

Despite the points I have just made, this book is not a book about theory—without a doubt the emphasis is on practical strategies for implementing a successful homework intervention program. To me, the real strength of this book is that it extends theory and provides clear and specific guidelines for practice within the homework context. I particularly appreciate both the breadth and depth with which Power and his colleagues address practice issues. That is, its scope (addressing interventions at the parent, teacher, and child levels) and detail (hands-on guidelines for practitioners) are impressive. It is a rare occasion to find an intervention model that is attentive to both *process* and *content* issues. Not only does this model consider "how to's" regarding homework interventions (the content), but it also includes practical considerations regarding clinically important issues (e.g., readiness for change, social validity, treatment integrity), group dynamics (e.g., "stubborn parents," oppositional children), and collaborative home–school consultation (i.e., Conjoint Behavioral Consultation [CBC], the process).

As Power, Karustis, and Habboushe indicate, many procedures for intervening with homework difficulties are available in the literature. However, the utility of many of these is determined largely by the ease with which practitioners can take what is presented and translate it into practice. The Homework Success Program is clearly unique in this regard. Screening instruments, intervention materials (forms, checklists, outlines), and outcome tools are provided, along with clear guidelines for their use. Further, pragmatic suggestions for "setting the stage," initiating the program, and involving children in a structured group intervention are clearly specified.

An extremely innovative aspect of the Homework Success Program is the application of a consultation model inclusive of home and school settings. Power and his colleagues have demonstrated nicely a novel extension of CBC (Sheridan, Kratochwill, & Bergan, 1996), which in this case allows ongoing home–school collaboration within the homework domain. Although collaboration has been suggested in the past (Olympia, Sheridan, & Jenson, 1994), no other homework intervention program effectively illustrates the manner in which home and school connections can be established. This program not only suggests the desirability of parents and teachers talking with each other but also provides important procedures for parents to prepare for the home–school meeting and how best to communicate with teachers.

DATA-BASED PERSPECTIVES

Another important aspect of the Homework Success Program is its empirically derived nature. The true benefits of any intervention program, regardless of its level of detail, are determined by its effects on the children and families served. "Best practices" concern the delivery of procedures that are likely to yield positive results based on research support. The procedures that together define the program (e.g., goal setting, reinforcement, parental involvement) are based on interventions that have been empirically supported and, importantly, demonstrated to be effective for use with children with ADHD.

True to the consultation process, the Homework Success Program allows for data-based evaluation of individual children's responsiveness to the intervention. Outcomes are assessed across several domains. The CBC process permits data-based monitoring and, if necessary, immediate and responsive adjustments of the environment, including antecedents (such as assignments given; nature, length, or difficulty of homework; homework environment; goals set for homework) and consequences (such as rewards delivered or grades earned). Parents and teachers collect data to evaluate success, with clear and simple outcome measures provided.

CONCLUSIONS

The goals and objectives of the Homework Success Program are broad and ambitious. They include positive effects on homework productivity, accuracy, and efficiency; knowledge about ADHD and behavior modification strategies; academic functioning; home–school relationships; family functioning; and self-esteem in children. Equally important but much less tangible is the somewhat concealed goal of this book: "to offer hope . . . for children and families coping with ADHD." It is my opinion that at least some of these benefits will result for most people involved in this program. If even one of these benefits ensue for the children, families, and teachers involved, the program will have succeeded.

As a researcher, clinician, and trainer, I can attest to the need for a resource such as *Homework Success for Children with ADHD*, and this book more than delivers. It is an understatement to say that as far as homework intervention programs go, *Homework Success for Children with ADHD* will be an invaluable resource for practitioners. It is a gem!

SUSAN M. SHERIDAN, PhD
University of Nebraska–Lincoln

REFERENCES

Bronfenbrenner, U. (1977). Toward an experimental ecology of human development. *American Psychologist, 32,* 513–531.

Olympia, D., Sheridan, S. M., & Jenson, W. R. (1994). Homework: A natural means of home–school collaboration. *School Psychology Quarterly, 9,* 60–80.

Sheridan, S. M., Kratochwill, T. R., & Bergan, J. R. (1996). *Conjoint Behavioral Consultation: A procedural manual.* New York: Plenum Press.

Preface: How to Use This Manual

This manual is intended for use by practitioners who are committed to assisting families in resolving significant homework difficulties. The manual is appropriate for a wide range of professionals, including school-based practitioners (e.g., school psychologists, guidance counselors, school social workers, school nurses), clinicians practicing in primary care health and mental health settings (e.g., psychologists, social workers, nurses, nurse practitioners, developmental and behavioral pediatricians), and clinicians providing services in tertiary care settings (e.g., psychologists, psychiatrists, social workers, nurses, nurse practitioners, and developmental and behavioral pediatricians). This manual is also intended for use by university-based trainers who are preparing students for careers as practitioners in educational, health, and behavioral health settings.

The Homework Success Program was designed to address the very challenging homework difficulties experienced by families coping with attention-deficit/hyperactivity disorder (ADHD) in a child. However, this program can be effective with families who do not have a child with ADHD but who experience significant problems with homework. Only minor adjustments in the program are needed to make it appropriate for families who are not coping with this disorder.

Homework Success is particularly appropriate for families with children enrolled in grades 1 through 6. Adaptations in this program may be needed to respond to the developmental issues of adolescents who are struggling with homework.

Homework Success was originally designed as a group intervention. This manual provides very specific guidelines for implementing the program in a group format with parents as well as with children. However, there are several additional ways in which this program can be used. Clinicians can adapt the procedures described in this manual and apply them with one family at a time. When it is not feasible to organize a group or when it appears that the family would not benefit from group intervention, clinicians can implement this program with a single family. In these cases, we recommend that the clinician follow the program in the sequential manner in which it is presented in this manual, albeit in a modified way that is responsive to the needs of the family.

An alternative way to use Homework Success, which may be appropriate for families who are already engaged in child and family counseling, is for clinicians to extract some of the components of Homework Success and incorporate them into their therapy. For example, at the outset of child and family counseling, the clinician and family may identify conduct problems, not homework problems, as the initial targets of intervention. During the course of counseling, however, the need to resolve homework problems may become paramount as a method to improve academic functioning and parent–child interactions. In situations in which the family has already received extensive training in behavioral strategies to address identified problems, clinicians may not feel that Homework Success components addressing positive reinforcement and punishment are needed. In these cases, it may be more appropriate to utilize the components of Homework Success that focus on facilitating collaborative home–school relationships and using behavioral strategies (e.g., establishing the homework routine, managing time and setting goals, and developing contingency contracts) that are unique to homework intervention.

Another way to adapt Homework Success is to use it as a source of potential intervention strategies when providing brief consultation to parents about homework problems. For example, when a child's homework problems are mild to moderate and the comprehensive Homework Success Program is not needed, a one- or two-session consultation with a clinician might be useful to the family. In these cases, strategies that address changing the homework routine and providing positive reinforcement for productive behavior may be very helpful. The use of more intensive strategies (e.g., time management and goal setting) or reductive techniques (e.g., response cost) may be less appropriate for a brief consultation.

Most of the chapters in this book present to practitioners highly specific guidelines for implementing the Homework Success Program. For example, there are chapters on recruiting and selecting participants, assessing intervention integrity and outcomes, setting up and initiating the program, conducting each of the six core sessions and a follow-up session, and conducting the child group concurrently with the parent group. Case illustrations from two groups of families who participated in Homework Success are also described.

The book also includes (in Chapter 2) an extensive review of the literature, which provides the theoretical and empirical support for the approaches used in this program. Given that the use of empirically supported strategies is necessary for successful intervention, we believe that an extensive review of the research literature pertaining to homework intervention is essential. Practitioners who are eager to implement this program can do so before they carefully read and reflect on the contents of Chapter 2. In these instances, practitioners may wish to read the conclusions at the end of Chapter 2 before implementing the program. However, we strongly recommend that clinicians return to Chapter 2 and read it carefully, so that they understand the theoretical and empirical foundation of Homework Success and can provide a convincing justification of the program to families, educators, and health service providers. University-based trainers who are using this manual to train students in behavioral family intervention will want to review Chapter 2 carefully to ensure that students fully understand the theoretical and empirical foundations of the program before attempting to implement it.

Contents

Homework Success
for Children with ADHD

## CHAPTER 1

Introduction to Homework Success

P roblems with homework are extremely common and often contribute to impairments in academic functioning. Students with attention-deficit/hyperactivity disorder (ADHD) are particularly prone to homework difficulties, given their intrinsic disorganization, forgetfulness, distractibility, lack of persistence, and carelessness. Many factors contribute to the academic skills deficits and underachievement commonly found in children with ADHD (DuPaul & Stoner, 1994); problems with the completion of homework assignments appear to be a primary contributor to the educational risk these youngsters face.

THE NEED FOR HOMEWORK INTERVENTION PROGRAMS FOR CHILDREN WITH ADHD

Homework is an important target of intervention for children with ADHD. Homework difficulties have pervasive effects on children and their families, including academic underachievement (Lahey et al., 1994), diminished self-esteem, conflictual parent–child relationships (Daniel, Power, Karustis, & Leff, 1999), and problems maintaining collaborative parent–teacher relationships (Buck et al., 1996). Increasing students' investment in homework and improving their productivity have been demonstrated to have positive effects, particularly with regard to gains in academic achievement (e.g., Cooper, Lindsay, Nye, & Greathouse, 1998; Paschal, Weinstein, & Walberg, 1984).

Given the substantial homework difficulties associated with ADHD, as well as the relationship between homework performance and academic outcomes, the need is apparent for a systematic homework program designed for children with ADHD. However, despite the availability of excellent behavioral intervention programs for children and adolescents with ADHD (see Barkley, 1998; DuPaul & Stoner, 1994), specialized intervention programs to address the homework difficulties of this population have not been developed sufficiently. Further, a number of excellent resources are available to assist clinicians in treating problems with homework (e.g., Anesko & Levine, 1987;

Olympia, Jenson, & Hepworth-Neville, 1996), but these programs typically have not been designed to address the unique needs of children with ADHD and their families.

PURPOSES OF THE HOMEWORK SUCCESS PROGRAM

The Homework Success Program was designed specifically to meet the homework-related needs of students with ADHD. Although the homework problems of children with ADHD are generally not unique, the difficulties they experience are often more severe and complex than those displayed by their peers. Also, research has shown that children with ADHD often require specialized instructional and behavioral interventions to address their educational needs and behavioral problems (DuPaul & Power, 2000; Pfiffner & Barkley, 1998). Nonetheless, this program can be very effective with students who have problems with homework but who do not meet criteria for this disorder. Families seeking to address the homework difficulties of children who do not have ADHD will also find this program to be helpful. In situations in which families are concerned about homework issues but in which the problems are relatively mild, involvement in the comprehensive Homework Success Program may not be needed. In these cases, brief consultation with a clinician may be sufficient. These strategies are described in detail in Chapters 6 through 9 of this manual.

Homework Success is a seven-session behavioral intervention program targeting problems specifically related to homework, especially those behaviors that are associated most closely with ADHD (e.g., remembering homework assignments, actively engaging in work assignments, persisting with work, using time efficiently). The program was designed in response to the frequently expressed concerns of primary caregivers and school professionals that homework problems rank among the most salient impairments experienced by children with ADHD. The program addresses a broad range of homework-related problems, given that children with ADHD tend to experience problems with homework from start to finish, including failing to adequately write down assignments, forgetting to bring home assignments, procrastinating and avoiding work, getting distracted easily and failing to persist with work, engaging in attention-getting strategies and arguing with parents, and neglecting to submit completed assignments.

The Homework Success Program is designed to address homework difficulties that arise in students in grades 1 through 6. We focus on children in the earlier grades given that this is the period in which parents and teachers begin to report substantial problems related to homework. During these grades it is critical to establish study skills and work habits that are fundamental to success later in school. Also, because the effects of homework problems are pervasive, often resulting in parenting stress and parent–child relationship problems, it is important to address these concerns as soon as they arise.

Students in grades 7 through 12 may also benefit from the strategies included in Homework Success. For example, the strategy of goal setting with contingency contracting may be very useful for older students with some modifications. However, Homework Success was specifically designed to be responsive to the developmental needs of the younger student. Students in the upper grades typically demand more autonomy and advance their positions more assertively than younger students. Although

Homework Success utilizes an approach that engages the child actively in planning and implementing interventions, the program may not offer older students sufficient autonomy and control in fashioning interventions to address their homework difficulties. As a result, if Homework Success is applied to adolescents without substantial modifications, it may evoke some degree of resistance from them. Students in the upper grades require an approach to intervention that is uniquely tailored to address their developmental needs. With older students, there typically needs to be a greater emphasis on developing parent–child communication skills, negotiating rules, developing behavioral contracts, and addressing the unique challenges of home–school collaboration when students have multiple teachers (Robin, 1998; Anesko & Levine, 1987).

The Homework Success Program can be very effective when applied in clinic settings, but it may be more useful and have a greater impact when applied in schools. With the reforms in health care in the 1990s resulting in a shift of service provision from clinic-based to community-based settings, the school increasingly is serving as a venue for the delivery of services for children and families (Nastasi, Varjas, Bernstein, & Pluymert, 1998). Advantages of a school-based model of service delivery include (1) the accessibility of schools to families living in the surrounding neighborhood; (2) the frequent opportunities for home–school collaboration; (3) the accessibility of naturalistic data that is very useful in progress monitoring and outcome assessment; (4) the cost effectiveness of services (Power, Atkins, Osborne, & Blum, 1994); and (5) the opportunities to provide services in a culturally sensitive, community-responsive manner (Manz, Power, Ginsburg-Block, & Dowrick, 2000).

The academic problems faced by many children with ADHD can frequently seem insurmountable. In this program it is our intention to offer hope, using approaches that have been empirically validated, for children and families coping with ADHD. Users of this manual can reasonably expect to achieve the following outcomes for families in their care who are attempting to manage ADHD-related problems:

- Increased understanding of ADHD and its relation to homework difficulties.
- Increased understanding of behavior modification principles and strategies.
- Improvement in the frequency and quality of home–school collaborations.
- Improvement in rates of homework completion and accuracy.
- Improvement in academic achievement.
- Improvement in parent–child relationships.
- Decreased parental stress.

CHAPTER 2

Background and Justification

Homework can be beneficial to the academic performance of students, but it is a challenging experience for many children and families. Children with ADHD and their parents, in particular, often encounter significant problems in the completion of homework assignments. This chapter presents the theoretical and empirical foundation for the Homework Success Program and reviews the literature in the following areas:

- The effects of homework on academic performance.
- The homework challenges experienced by children with ADHD.
- Empirically supported interventions for improving homework performance.
- The importance of a comprehensive approach to intervention.
- The need to systemically monitor adherence with intervention procedures.
- The importance of multimethod outcome assessment.
- Strategies to improve intervention adherence.
- Guidelines for combining medication with behavioral intervention.
- The importance of follow-up services.

EFFECTS OF HOMEWORK ON ACADEMIC PERFORMANCE

Homework is defined as assignments given by teachers that are to be performed by students outside of school or during noninstructional classroom time (Cooper, 1989; Keith & DeGraff, 1997). Homework assignments can be classified into four categories: (1) practice assignments, designed to review material presented in class; (2) preparation assignments, designed to prepare students for topics that will be presented in class in the near future; (3) extension homework, which facilitates the generalization of concepts from familiar to unfamiliar contexts; and (4) creative assignments, which require the integration of knowledge and concepts to create a novel product (Lee & Pruitt, 1979). When students are in the elementary grades, homework is typically designed to practice skills or to prepare for future lessons. Homework given to middle school and high school students typically includes assignments from each category, including homework designed to develop conceptual understanding and the ability to apply knowledge to novel situations.

Studies regarding the effectiveness of homework generally support the popular notion that homework has positive effects on academic grades and test scores (Cooper, 1989; Keith et al., 1993). Research indicates that students who are assigned homework perform at a higher level than those who are not and that amount of time spent on homework is positively correlated with academic achievement (Keith & DeGraff, 1997). Further, recent research has indicated that amount of homework completed is more strongly related to academic outcomes than is amount of time spent on homework (Cooper et al., 1998).

The effectiveness of homework appears to vary as a function of student grade level. High school students have repeatedly demonstrated a positive relationship between time spent on homework and academic achievement (Foyle, 1984; Keith & Benson, 1992). Although the positive effects of homework on middle school and elementary school students have also been shown (Keith et al., 1993), research suggests that the magnitude of the effect of homework on academic achievement is somewhat lower in the elementary and middle school years (Cooper, 1989).

Although the direct effects of homework on academic performance appear relatively modest in the elementary years, there are additional benefits to assigning homework to young students. Homework may help to develop study skills and work habits, which can be useful to students in the classroom and during homework when they get older (Keith & DeGraff, 1997). Also, homework provides frequent opportunities for home–school collaboration and parental involvement in school (Olympia, Sheridan, & Jenson, 1994), which have been shown to be strongly related to student outcomes (Christenson, Rounds, & Franklin, 1992; Fantuzzo, Davis, & Ginsburg, 1995).

THE HOMEWORK PROBLEMS OF CHILDREN WITH ADHD

ADHD is characterized by problems with inattention and/or hyperactivity-impulsivity that result in significant levels of impairment in academic or social functioning (American Psychiatric Association, 1994). This disorder is now delineated into three subtypes, including ADHD, predominantly inattentive type; ADHD, predominantly hyperactive-impulsive type; and ADHD, combined type (see Table 2.1).

Research has repeatedly affirmed the distinction between the inattentive and combined subtypes; studies are needed to validate the hyperactive–impulsive subtype (Power & DuPaul, 1996). ADHD has been shown to be more prevalent in boys than girls, with the ratio estimated to be about 3:1 (Barkley, 1998; Power, Andrews et al., 1998; Szatmari, Offord, & Boyle, 1989). Approximately 25% of children with ADHD have learning disabilities, including reading, math, and/or writing disorders. Regardless of whether they have learning disabilities, a strong majority underachieve academically (DuPaul & Stoner, 1994). Children with the inattentive subtypes of ADHD (ADHD, inattentive type; ADHD, combined type) appear to be particularly at risk for

TABLE 2.1. Diagnostic Criteria for Attention-Deficit/Hyperactivity Disorder (ADHD)

A. Either (1) or (2):

    (1) six (or more) of the following symptoms of **inattention** have persisted for at least 6 months to a degree that is maladaptive and inconsistent with developmental level:

        Inattention
        (a) often fails to give close attention to details or makes careless mistakes in schoolwork, work, or other activities
        (b) often has difficulty sustaining attention in tasks or play activities
        (c) often does not seem to listen when spoken to directly
        (d) often does not follow through on instructions and fails to finish schoolwork, chores, or duties in the workplace (not due to oppositional behavior or failure to understand instructions)
        (e) often has difficulty organizing tasks and activities
        (f) often avoids, dislikes, or is reluctant to engage in tasks that require sustained mental effort (such as schoolwork or homework)
        (g) often loses things necessary for tasks or activities (e.g., toys, school assignments, pencils, books, or tools)
        (h) is often easily distracted by extraneous stimuli
        (i) is often forgetful in daily activities

    (2) six (or more) of the following symptoms of **hyperactivity–impulsivity** have persisted for at least 6 months to a degree that is maladaptive and inconsistent with developmental level:

        Hyperactivity
        (a) often fidgets with hands or feet or squirms in seat
        (b) often leaves seat in classroom or in other situations in which remaining seated is expected
        (c) often runs about or climbs excessively in situations in which it is inappropriate (in adolescents or adults, may be limited to subjective feelings of restlessness)
        (d) often has difficulty playing or engaging in leisure activities quietly is often "on the go" or often acts as if "driven by a motor"
        (f) often talks excessively

        Impulsivity
        (g) often blurts out answers before questions have been completed
        (h) often has difficulty awaiting turn
        (i) often interrupts or intrudes on others (e.g., butts into conversations or games)

B. Some hyperactive–impulsive or inattentive symptoms that caused impairment were present before age 7 years.

C. Some impairment from the symptoms is present in two or more settings (e.g., at school [or work] and at home).

D. There must be clear evidence of clinically significant impairment in social, academic, or occupational functioning

E. The symptoms do not occur exclusively during the course of Pervasive Developmental Disorder, Schizophrenia, or other Psychotic Disorder and are not better accounted for by another mental disorder (e.g., Mood Disorder, Anxiety Disorder, or a Personality Disorder).

(cont.)

TABLE 2.1. *(cont.)*

Code based on type:

314.01 **Attention-Deficit/Hyperactivity Disorder, Combined Type:** if both Criteria A1 and A2 are met for the past 6 months

314.00 **Attention-Deficit/Hyperactivity Disorder, Predominantly Inattentive Type:** if Criterion A1 is met but Criterion A2 is not met for the past 6 months

314.01 **Attention-Deficit/Hyperactivity Disorder, Predominantly Hyperactive–Impulsive Type:** if Criterion A2 is met but Criterion A1 is not met for the past 6 months

Note. From American Psychiatric Association (1994). Copyright 1994 by the American Psychiatric Association. Reprinted by permission.

cognitive impairment, academic underachievement, and homework problems (Lahey et al., 1994).

The academic problems of children with ADHD are related to multiple variables, but two factors appear particularly important. First, children with ADHD are less actively engaged in academic instruction than their classmates without ADHD. Children with ADHD typically display significantly lower rates of on-task behavior and engaged time during instruction and classroom work than their peers (Abikoff, Gittelman-Klein, Klein, 1977). The academic disengagement of children with ADHD places them at a significant disadvantage academically: A substantial amount of research has demonstrated the strong relationship between level of academic engaged time and academic achievement (see Shapiro, 1996).

Second, students with attention and learning problems require more instruction and practice than their peers to keep pace in the classroom (Zentall, 1993). Unfortunately, educational systems often are not prepared to provide these students with the additional instruction and practice they need (Landrum, Al-Mateen, Ellis, Singh, & Ricketts, 1993). Further, families are often not equipped to support children who are highly disorganized (Kay, Fitzgerald, Paradee, & Mellencamp, 1994). Thus, to improve the academic functioning of students with attention and learning problems, it is necessary to (1) improve their on-task behavior and engagement in academic work, and (2) provide them with more opportunities to learn and practice academic skills (Mercugliano, Power, & Blum, 1999). Homework provides children innumerable opportunities to learn and practice academic skills. Assisting children to take advantage of these opportunities by becoming more actively engaged in their work can be a very useful learning strategy.

Although surprisingly little research has investigated the homework difficulties of children with ADHD, it is clear that a majority of these children display more frequent and severe homework problems than their peers (Karustis, Power, Rescorla, Eiraldi, & Gallagher, 1998; Lahey et al., 1994). Children with ADHD frequently display the following types of problems: failure to write down homework assignments, failure to bring home assignments, unwillingness to begin work at the designated time, lack of persistence, distractibility, failure to complete work, conflict with parents, carelessness, and failure to return assignments to the teacher.

INTERVENTIONS TO IMPROVE HOMEWORK PERFORMANCE

Several interventions have been designed to improve homework performance, including rates of completion and accuracy, as well as efficiency. These interventions can be subdivided into those focused on antecedents and those pertaining to the consequences of homework. In the Homework Success Program, changing antecedents is emphasized at the outset during the initiation of the program and during the first two sessions (see Chapters 6, 7, and 8, this volume). Modifying consequences is the focus of the third, fourth, and fifth sessions (see Chapters 9, 10, and 11).

Antecedents

The antecedents of homework are a broad range of variables and situations that set the stage for doing homework. A critical school-based factor that can affect homework performance is the assignment given by the teacher. Homework that has a specific purpose, is closely related to classroom instruction, and generates a product appears to be beneficial for students (Keith & DeGraff, 1997). Assignments that are designed to practice skills learned in the classroom should be able to be completed with high rates of accuracy, exceeding the 90% level (Gickling & Thompson, 1985). Practice assignments should be limited in length, and the teacher should attempt to vary the types of assignments given (Keith & DeGraff, 1997). Further, for homework to be effective, assignments must be clearly stated, and provisions must be made for the student to take thorough, accurate notes of work assigned (Anesko & Levine, 1987).

Parents clearly have a very important role in creating an environment that is suitable for doing homework. A key strategy is to establish a regular time for homework that takes into consideration fluctuations in the child's ability to pay attention and the parents' ability to carefully monitor behavior during after-school hours (Olympia, Jenson, Clark, & Sheridan, 1992). Another critical component is to establish a place for homework that minimizes distractions, such as television and the play of siblings, and promotes attention to task (Olympia et al., 1992). Further, it is important for parents to offer instructions in a clear, concise manner.

Consequences

The consequences of homework are the various ways that parents, teachers, peers, siblings, and children themselves respond to the behaviors emitted during homework. Teacher responses to homework can have a significant effect on performance. Grading homework and providing feedback very shortly after assignments are submitted have been shown to have a positive effect on achievement (Paschal et al., 1984). Home–school notes, whereby the teacher informs parents on a daily basis about the homework performance of a student, have been shown to be effective (Kelley, 1990; Lordeman &

Winett, 1980). Further, peers can serve an important role in the completion of homework. Peer-mediated strategies that involve teams of students working on homework assignments and group contingencies have been shown to be effective in improving homework performance (Olympia, Sheridan, Jenson, & Andrews, 1994).

A wealth of research has demonstrated the impact that parents can have on the attention and behavior of children (Kazdin, 1997). Parent training has been demonstrated to be a very effective method for helping parents to change their behavior and to achieve desired, targeted goals for their child (Forehand & McMahon, 1981). One of the hallmarks of parenting programs is training parents to selectively attend to and reinforce responsible, productive child behavior and to ignore and refrain from reinforcing nonadaptive, unproductive behaviors (McMahon, Forehand, & Griest, 1981). Other critical components include training parents to effectively deliver requests for compliance and providing specific labels when issuing verbal praise (Forehand & Scarboro, 1975). Enhanced reinforcement programs that involve the provision of tokens and concrete reinforcers for the attainment of targeted goals have been shown to be effective in improving behavior and performance (Anesko & O'Leary, 1982). Because the value of a reinforcer typically declines with repeated use, particularly with children who have ADHD, it is very important that reinforcers be varied on a frequent basis. Procedures that vary reinforcers and involve an element of uncertainty, such as the "mystery motivator" technique, have been demonstrated to be very effective in improving homework performance (Moore, Waguespack, Wickstrom, Witt, & Gaydos, 1994).

The systematic withdrawal of positive reinforcement through the use of response cost and time-out procedures can be very useful in changing children's behavior (Forehand & McMahon, 1981). Response cost is often used in the context of a token reinforcement system and involves the removal of points or tokens when specified undesirable behaviors are committed by the child (Barkley, 1997). Time-out refers to the systematic removal of a child from opportunities to receive positive reinforcement, which is usually operationalized as the placement of a child onto a chair in a quiet, nonstimulating location at home or in school. Time-out can be a highly effective intervention when it is used as an immediate response to targeted behaviors and results in a significant loss of positive reinforcement. Time-out is often ineffective when it enables the child to avoid a demanding task, such as homework (Shriver & Allen, 1996). In this case, time-out may actually serve to negatively reinforce avoidant, unproductive behavior (DuPaul & Ervin, 1996; Northup et al., 1995). For this reason, parents need to be extremely careful in using time-out in addressing problems that arise with homework. Given that children with ADHD typically avoid tasks that require sustained effort, time-out is rarely an effective response to unproductive behavior with these individuals.

A particularly promising approach to the behavioral treatment of homework problems is goal setting with contingency contracting (Kahle & Kelley, 1994; Miller & Kelley, 1994). This strategy consists of training a parent and child to (1) establish realistic goals for homework completion, accuracy, and duration; (2) evaluate performance in relation to established goals; and (3) administer positive reinforcers, using a menu of reinforcers negotiated by the parent and child, contingent on the child's attainment of goals. This strategy was demonstrated to be superior to a standard parent training intervention in improving parent-ratings of homework performance, as well as children's actual performance on homework assignments (Kahle & Kelley, 1994). These results strongly suggest that goal setting with contingency contracting should be a major component of a comprehensive homework intervention program (see Chapter 10, this volume).

A specific problem with homework can have multiple purposes or functions that vary from family to family. For example, getting out of a seat during homework can serve the purpose of eliciting parental involvement and attention, but it can also enable the child to escape work and secure negative reinforcement for unproductive behavior (DuPaul & Ervin, 1996). For these reasons, it is important that homework interventions be tailored to the needs of each child and family (DuPaul, Eckert, & McGoey, 1997). One way to help parents analyze the functions of homework behavior is to train them to recognize and record the antecedents and consequences of the specific problems that arise during homework.

PARENT-TRAINING PROGRAMS FOR HOMEWORK PROBLEMS

Many parent-training programs have been developed to improve the homework performance of children. Examples of these programs include Winning the Homework War (Anesko & Levine, 1987), Homework without Tears (Canter & Hausner, 1987), and Sanity Savers for Parents: Tips for Tackling Homework (Olympia et al., 1996). Most of these programs present useful interventions that involve modifying both the antecedents and the consequences of homework behavior.

Although many of these parent-training programs are based on sound principles of instruction and behavior management and incorporate intervention components that have been empirically demonstrated to be effective, they have some limitations, particularly for the treatment of children with ADHD. First, these programs were designed for students with homework problems but not specifically for children with ADHD. The short attention span, lack of persistence, and disorganization that is typical of children with ADHD very often result in homework problems that are significant and contribute to substantial academic impairment and highly conflictual parent–child interactions. Children with ADHD respond well to behavioral treatments, but they often require specialized interventions to address their problems (DuPaul & Stoner, 1994). Second, most of these programs focus solely on the training of parents and do not incorporate the child and teachers into the treatment in a meaningful way. Offering a more comprehensive program that involves the child and teachers in the planning and implementation of interventions can be extremely useful and may augment the benefits of parent-training programs (Weiner, Sheridan, & Jenson, 1998). Third, most parent-training programs fail to monitor carefully the integrity with which the interventions are being implemented. As a result, it is often unclear whether the interventions are being implemented as intended. Fourth, there is very little empirical support for the effectiveness of these programs (Olympia, Sheridan, & Jenson, 1994). Most of these programs have not been systematically evaluated using multimethod assessment measurement procedures. Notable exceptions are single-case research studies conducted by Rhoades and Kratochwill (1998), as well as by Weiner et al. (1998).

Parent-training programs can be provided to individual sets of parents or to groups. An advantage of the group format is that it provides opportunities for parents to support each other, which can be very helpful given the stress and isolation that many parents of children with ADHD experience (Barkley, 1998). Because parents who are stressed often have significant problems using behavioral strategies effectively (Wahler & Dumas, 1989), creating a context within which they can derive emotional support from other parents may help them to be more effective in using behavioral techniques. Group parent training also provides a forum for problem solving through which parents can derive useful, practical suggestions from their peers for addressing homework problems at home. A further advantage is the cost effectiveness of groups.

NEED FOR SPECIALIZED INTERVENTIONS FOR ADHD

Children with ADHD respond very well to instructional and behavioral interventions, but they generally require more intensive treatment than their peers to accomplish significant behavioral change. For example, selective attention, which involves the strategic use of verbal praise for productive, compliant behavior and ignoring for unproductive, uncooperative behavior, is often effective in changing the behavior of children with mild attention and behavior problems, but it is often not sufficient for children with ADHD. Youngsters with this disorder often require enhanced reinforcement systems, which may involve the use of token systems, to accomplish a significant level of change (Pfiffner & O'Leary, 1993; see also Chapter 9, this volume). Also, systems of behavior modification that use positive reinforcement alone, although desirable, are generally not sufficient to address the attention and behavior problems of children with ADHD. For this reason, strategies that involve the strategic use of punishment, such as corrective feedback and response cost, are often important to include in an intervention program for children with ADHD (DuPaul & Power, 2000; Pfiffner & Barkley, 1998; see also Chapter 11, this volume). Further, because children with ADHD habituate to situations quickly and require high levels of novelty to maintain interest and attention (Zentall & Dwyer, 1988), it is important to vary reinforcers frequently when using behavior modification systems with these individuals.

INCLUDING TEACHERS IN HOMEWORK PROGRAMS

The teacher serves a critical role in the design and completion of homework assignments. Teachers determine (1) which of the four types of homework to assign, (2) the congruence of homework with classroom instruction, (3) the level of difficulty of homework, and (4) the amount of homework to be assigned. Teachers also determine whether and how homework is evaluated and the immediacy of homework feedback, both of which can have an effect on performance (Paschal et al., 1984). In addition, homework can provide an opportunity for teachers to promote an effective partnership with parents (Olympia, Sheridan, & Jenson, 1994). Through this collaboration teachers can invite parents to become increasingly involved in their child's education, which in itself can contribute to better student outcomes (Epstein, 1991; Fantuzzo et al., 1995).

Sheridan and colleagues (Sheridan, Kratochwill, & Bergan, 1996, 1997) have developed a model of home–school collaboration, known as Conjoint Behavioral Consultation (CBC), that applies the principles of behavioral consultation to resolve school-related problems. This model has been used as a foundation for intervention programs to improve children's homework performance (see Weiner et al., 1998). Their approach to resolving homework difficulties consists of involving parents and teachers in a partnership to (1) identify problems, (2) analyze the nature and function of each problem, (3) plan and implement intervention approaches, and (4) evaluate effectiveness and make modifications in the intervention plan as needed (Sheridan et al., 1996). Clinicians guide parents and teachers to design interventions similar to those previously described. Parents and teachers are encouraged to modify and streamline the procedures to make them more meaningful and acceptable to them. The CBC model provides a very useful framework for constructing a comprehensive homework intervention program and is an important part of the foundation for the Homework Success Program. Strategies for operationalizing the CBC model are embedded in Homework Success, but there is particular emphasis on this approach during the initiation of the program and after Session 4 (see Chapters 6 and 10).

INCLUDING THE CHILD IN HOMEWORK PROGRAMS

Parent-training programs typically do not involve children directly in the intervention. Parents are assigned the challenging task of explaining new approaches to children, negotiating behavioral contracts with them, and eliciting their child's cooperation. Many parents, particularly those who have children with ADHD who may be defiant, will have significant problems negotiating with their child and gaining their child's compliance (Barkley, 1998). The process of intervention is often facilitated by introducing children to the principles and strategies their parents are learning in parent training and by inviting the child to participate in designing strategies. In fact, a body of research is accumulating that demonstrates that programs that involve both parents and children in the intervention process are more effective than approaches that work with parents or the child alone (Frankel, Myatt, Cantwell, & Feinberg, 1997; Webster-Stratton & Hammond, 1997). For this reason, we strongly recommend that clinicians actively involve children in the Homework Success Program (see Chapter 14).

MONITORING INTERVENTION INTEGRITY

A key to successful intervention is to ensure that treatments are applied as intended, a procedure that has been referred to as intervention integrity (Gresham, 1989; Moncher & Prinz, 1991). Interventions that have been demonstrated through research to be effective often are not successful in actual practice because treatment techniques are not applied as designed. Parent-training programs typically outline specific guidelines for clinicians to follow in implementing interventions, but they may fail to include procedures for monitoring treatment integrity.

Numerous strategies have been developed to facilitate the monitoring of intervention integrity. These techniques include (1) use of scripts to prompt the clinician to follow specific steps of intervention, (2) self-monitoring adherence by recording on written scripts whether each intervention step has been accomplished, and (3) direct observation of sessions with the provision of feedback by expert clinicians (Ehrhardt, Barnett, Lentz, Stollar, & Reifin, 1996; Power, Dowrick, Ginsburg-Block, & Manz, 2000). The use of scripts to facilitate intervention integrity has been found to be very useful in facilitating successful intervention. We recommend the use of each of these procedures in monitoring the integrity with which Homework Success interventions are implemented (see Chapter 4).

EVALUATING INTERVENTION OUTCOME

Homework difficulties have pervasive effects on children and families, including (1) reduced rates of homework completion and accuracy (Miller & Kelley, 1991), (2) impairments in academic functioning (Cooper, 1989; Keith & DeGraff, 1997), and (3) conflictual parent–child interactions (Anesko, Schoiock, Ramirez, & Levine, 1987). When evaluating the outcomes of a homework intervention program, it is important to assess its impact in each of these domains.

Various types of measurement procedures are available to evaluate the effectiveness of intervention programs that address homework problems, including parent reports, teacher reports, child self-reports, homework samples collected during baseline and intervention conditions, and records of homework kept by the teacher. Each of these methods has advantages and limitations. For example, parent reports of homework can be very useful in that parents can provide very specific information about homework because of the innumerable opportunities they have to observe their child. A limitation of parent reports is their lack of objectivity, in that parents are often a primary agent of change in homework intervention programs. Homework samples have the advantage of providing objective information about the child, but these data do not provide information about child, family, and school variables that may be contributing to homework difficulties.

Because each type of measure provides a unique set of information about homework and because of the limitations of each type of assessment procedure, it is very important to use a multimethod assessment battery in evaluating the effects of a homework intervention program. The Homework Success Program includes the following measurement procedures for evaluating outcome: (1) parent reports of homework productivity and time spent doing homework, (2) teacher reports of academic performance, (3) parent and child reports of family interactions, (4) homework samples scored for rates of completion and accuracy, (5) classwork samples scored for rates of completion and accuracy, and (6) teacher records of homework performance and academic achievement (see Chapter 4).

Because homework problems are difficult to resolve and tend to re-emerge over time, particularly with children who have ADHD, it is important to assess outcomes over extended periods of time. Follow-up assessment can determine the long-term benefits of the program for a child and family, but more important, it can identify problems that reemerge over time, thus signaling the need for additional intervention.

IMPROVING INTERVENTION ADHERENCE

Behaviorally oriented parent-training programs such as Homework Success have been demonstrated to be effective in treating the problems associated with ADHD (Anastopoulos, Shelton, DuPaul, & Guevremont, 1993; Dubey, O'Leary, & Kaufman, 1983; Pisterman et al., 1989). Unfortunately, up to 50% of families do not follow through with recommendations made by clinicians for counseling and parent training (Bennett, Power, Rostain, & Carr, 1996; Joost, Chessare, Schaeufele, Link, & Weaver, 1989), and about 50% of families who enter psychological treatment prematurely terminate intervention (Brown, Borden, Wynne, Spunt, & Clingerman, 1987; Firestone & Witt, 1982). Low socioeconomic status, high levels of marital conflict, single parenthood, parental depression, and parental sense of isolation have been associated with relatively poor adherence to parent-training programs (Dumas & Wahler, 1983; Firestone & Witt, 1982; Kazdin, 1997).

Prochaska and colleagues have developed a model that is useful in understanding how individuals change (see Prochaska, DiClemente, & Norcross, 1992; Prochaska et al., 1994). According to Prochaska, for individuals to change, they must be ready and willing to do so. He posits five stages of readiness for change:

1. *Precontemplation,* which refers to a lack of intention to change behavior, primarily because of failure to recognize that there is a problem.
2. *Contemplation,* the stage in which individuals are aware that there is a problem and are assessing whether the investment of time, energy, and financial resources needed to achieve a solution is worthwhile.
3. *Preparation,* referring to an intention to take action and a commitment to take action in the near future.
4. *Action,* the stage in which individuals actively invest in the interventions needed to accomplish behavioral change.
5. *Maintenance,* the stage in which individuals work toward consolidating treatment gains and preventing relapse.

In order for families to benefit from behaviorally oriented parent-training programs, they must be in the preparation or action stages of the change process.

The decision to actively invest in intervention involves assessing the benefits to be attained by changing behavior as opposed to the costs involved in treatment (Prochaska et al., 1994). Numerous factors have an impact on how families analyze the benefits and costs of intervention and whether they are able to successfully move through the contemplation and preparation phases so that they are ready to begin intervention. Two critical considerations are the social validity and the feasibility of the interventions. Social validity refers to perceptions that consumers of an intervention approach have about the appropriateness and fairness of the goals, strategies, and outcomes of intervention (Schwartz & Baer, 1991). The effectiveness of intervention depends in part on whether families and professionals share the same goals, endorse the same set of intervention strategies, and agree on the outcomes of treatment. In general, parents and teachers prefer behavioral as opposed to pharmacological methods of intervention, view positive reinforcement procedures as more acceptable than punitive techniques, and prefer brief, relatively simple interventions over more complex and time-consuming approaches (Brown & Sawyer, 1998; Liu, Robin, Brenner, & Eastman, 1991; Power, Hess, & Bennett, 1995).

Several factors mediate consumers' perceptions about the social validity of intervention, including the severity of the problem (Elliott, 1988); knowledge of the problem or disorder being treated (Bennett et al., 1996); involvement of the child in decision making (Brown & Sawyer, 1998); the extent to which systematic procedures are used to assess outcomes (Aman & Wolford, 1995); and the effects of intervention on the child, family, teacher, and peers (Reimers, Wacker, & Koeppl, 1987).

Feasibility refers to the convenience and accessibility of resources for providing intervention. Clinic-based programs pose significant challenges to parents, including high costs for services, distance from home, scheduling problems, and transportation costs (Cunningham, Bremner, & Boyle, 1995; Power et al., 1994). The shift to managed care has presented additional impediments to service delivery, in particular restricting access to a sizable proportion of behavioral health providers.

Families from urban settings often face the most significant challenges in gaining access to the services they need, due in part to economic factors that restrict access to care. In addition, urban families, particularly those belonging to minority groups, typically display different patterns of help-seeking behavior than suburban, white families. For example, African American families often will seek help within the neighborhood from their families or religious communities before they will consider going to a clinic (McMiller & Weisz, 1996). The reluctance of minority families to seek help in clinical settings may be related in part to a concern that professionals may not be responsive to cultural factors that influence their thinking and behavior (Comer & Haynes, 1991; Garbarino & Abramowitz, 1992).

The literature on readiness for change, social validity, and feasibility suggests that the following practices may be useful in assisting families to become ready for intervention programs such as Homework Success:

1. Assess each family's readiness for change and enroll a family in the intervention program only when they are ready for this level of commitment (see Chapter 3).
2. Assess parents', children's, and teachers' perceptions of the social validity of program interventions before and during the course of treatment and make modifications in intervention strategies accordingly (see Chapter 4).
3. Educate parents and teachers about the problem and interventions that have been shown to be effective in resolving the problem (see Chapter 6).

4. Engage the parents, child, and teachers in a collaborative process to plan interventions (see Chapter 6).
5. Assess outcome systematically (see Chapter 4).

For families from urban settings, community-based approaches to intervention, such as establishing parent-training programs in schools, churches, and community settings, may improve access to care and involvement by families (Cunningham & Cunningham, 1998). Also, establishing members of the community in leadership roles may enhance the effectiveness of parent training. In urban settings, clinicians who conduct parent-training programs often do not understand the cultural backgrounds of the families they serve, which may reduce the effectiveness of the service. Enlisting, training, and empowering community residents to serve as cofacilitators in parent-training programs may improve the cultural sensitivity and community responsiveness of this approach to intervention (Dowrick et al., in press; Manz et al., 2000).

DEVELOPING A PLAN FOR MEDICATION

In general, the most effective intervention for children with ADHD is stimulant medication, including methylphenidate, dextroamphetamine, pemoline, and Adderall (Klein & Abikoff, 1997; Pelham et al., 1993). An estimated 70–80% of children demonstrate marked gains in attention and behavior in response to stimulant medication (DuPaul, Barkley, & Connor, 1998). Stimulants are generally very safe, and only a small percentage of children who take this medication will experience side effects of sufficient magnitude to preclude treatment (Barkley, McMurray, Edelbrock, & Robbins, 1990). For these reasons, most families of children with ADHD should give serious consideration to using stimulant medication.

Despite its effectiveness, medication is not a cure for ADHD, and it is not sufficient to manage the major problems associated with this disorder (DuPaul & Rapport, 1993). Academic and behavioral interventions are often needed as a supplement to or instead of medication to address the academic problems of these youngsters. Given that the use of stimulant medication may be problematic during after-school hours because it may keep children awake in the evening, specialized instructional and behavioral interventions are particularly important during homework.

Although medication can be very effective in addressing the academic and behavior problems of children with ADHD, a problem arises when families introduce this intervention during the course of a behavioral intervention program such as Homework Success. Stimulant medication often has such strong effects on attention and behavior that it can become difficult to differentiate whether treatment gains are due to the Homework Success Program or to medication. For this reason, we typically recommend that families refrain from initiating a trial of medication during the course of homework intervention. Families are encouraged to introduce medication either before Homework Success begins or after the seven-session intervention has been completed.

SUSTAINING THE COURSE OF INTERVENTION

ADHD is a chronic disorder whose effects typically endure into adolescence and often into adulthood (Weiss & Hechtman, 1993). Interventions for ADHD, including medication and behavior therapies, are usually effective, but only when they are being actively applied. There is very little evidence to indicate that the effects of treatments for ADHD persist after the interventions have been terminated (Barkley, 1998). For this reason, it is very important that brief interventions such as Homework Success include follow-up sessions to help families maintain treatment effects and prevent relapse (Barkley, 1997; Prochaska et al., 1992; see also Chapter 13, this volume). When feasible, it is useful to monitor outcomes long after the intensive period of treatment has concluded, so that families and professionals can see when impairments are beginning to reemerge and when the family needs to engage again in intervention.

CONCLUSIONS

The literature reviewed in this chapter supports the following conclusions with regard to providing a specialized program of homework intervention for children with ADHD:

1. Homework is an important target of intervention because it has direct effects on academic achievement, as well as indirect effects on educational functioning, by fostering collaborative home–school relationships and building study skills.

2. Children with attention and learning problems, including those with ADHD, need very frequent opportunities to learn and practice academic skills to keep pace with their peers. Homework can provide these children with additional opportunities to learn and practice skills. Effective homework interventions can help these children to take better advantage of the opportunities provided to them through homework.

3. Behavioral interventions are effective in addressing homework difficulties. Behavioral interventions that include strategies to address the antecedents and consequences of homework behavior have the greatest probability of being effective.

4. Most children with ADHD require specialized behavioral interventions to address their problems with homework. These strategies include environmental changes to promote productive behavior, token reinforcement systems, frequent variations in positive reinforcers, and the strategic use of punishment techniques such as corrective feedback and response cost. Time-out should be used sparingly during homework, particularly for children with ADHD, because of its potential to inadvertently reinforce unproductive, task-avoidant behavior.

5. Goal setting with contingency contracting is a powerful tool in a homework intervention program. This strategy fosters collaboration between the parents and child to achieve important homework goals.

6. Homework interventions need to be tailored to meet the needs of each child and family. Homework problems vary in their form and function. Effective programs of

intervention train parents and children to assess the function of homework difficulties by assessing both the antecedents and consequences of behavior.

7. Parent training is an effective method of improving homework performance.

8. Including teachers in a homework intervention program is important because they have the ability to determine the type and amount of homework assigned to students. Also, teachers can improve homework performance by providing salient feedback as soon as possible after homework is submitted.

9. Including the child in a homework program is important because interventions are more likely to be effective and acceptable to families when the child is involved.

10. Monitoring intervention integrity is essential in delivering a homework intervention service. Having clinicians self-monitor performance using written scripts is a useful tool to ensure integrity. Also, direct observation of sessions with specific feedback provided by experts can help to improve treatment integrity.

11. Homework intervention programs should be evaluated carefully using multimethod evaluation batteries administered before, during, and after intervention, as well as periodically during follow-up. These batteries should include information provided by multiple sources, including the parent, teacher, and child. Outcome should be assessed with regard to changes in homework completion and accuracy, academic functioning, and parent–child interaction.

12. Homework intervention programs should include strategies to improve adherence with treatment. It is critical that services are (a) provided to families when they are ready to make a commitment to treatment, (b) offered in a venue that is readily accessible to families, (c) delivered in a culturally responsive manner, (d) designed in collaboration with the parents and child, and (e) modified periodically in response to feedback from family members and teachers about intervention acceptability.

13. Medication, in particular the stimulants, serves an important role in the treatment of problems related to ADHD, which may include homework issues. Medicating children during homework can be problematic for some children in that a common side effect is insomnia.

14. Because of the chronic nature of ADHD, it is important that outcomes are monitored for a sustained period after the intensive stage of intervention has been completed. When problems arise, it is important to provide follow-up services tailored to meet the needs of the child and family.

## CHAPTER 3

Recruiting and Screening Participants

For the Homework Success Program to be effective, it is essential that clinicians carefully recruit and select participants. As a leading authority on group intervention programs noted years ago, "the fate of a therapy group . . . is to a large extent determined before the first group session" (Yalom, 1975, p. 19). Most important, delineation of criteria for participation in groups has been found to be associated with increased rates of attendance, retention of instructional content, and engagement in the group process (Piper & Perrault, 1989).

This chapter includes a discussion of the following: (1) guidelines for informing referral sources and families about Homework Success; (2) special considerations for recruiting participants; (3) criteria for identifying families who are likely to benefit from the program; and (4) procedures for assisting families whose needs cannot be adequately addressed by this program.

RECRUITING PARTICIPANTS FOR CLINICAL SETTINGS

A wide range of professionals may be interested in referring families to a program like Homework Success. The following is a description of methods to inform each of these groups of professionals about this program.

Physicians and Behavioral Health Professionals as Referring Agents

Primary care pediatric providers and behavioral health professionals are important to Homework Success, both as sources of referrals and as collaborators in the screening, assessment, and intervention process. Appendix A in this volume includes both a sample letter and an information flyer that can be sent to these referring agents. Clinicians intending to conduct the Homework Success Program need to provide information to referring agents that specifies the key elements of the program, as well as criteria for participation. As the sample letter and flyer make clear, clinicians should be available to referral sources and potential participants for questions.

School Professionals as Referring Agents

If Homework Success is to be conducted in a clinic setting, we recommend that the clinician inform school personnel from surrounding school districts. For public schools, we suggest that the initial contact be with the coordinator of pupil personnel services or special education services. Proceeding in this manner will enable the clinician to secure proper authorization from the school to recruit families for the program. This can be accomplished by sending a letter to the coordinator (see Appendix A). For private schools, the principal should be contacted directly.

With proper authorization from a school official, group leaders can proceed to contact other school personnel. We suggest that an introductory and recruitment letter that is similar to those previously discussed be issued to the Child Study Team (CST) coordinator, counselor, or school psychologist (see Appendix A). This letter will inform the recipient about the Homework Success Program, and request assistance in recruiting participants. Many CST coordinators, counselors, and school psychologists will wish to refer families to the program themselves. A letter addressed to parents can be used to inform parents about Homework Success and to request them to consider enrollment in this program (see Appendix A). In some cases, with the authorization of the principal, it may be appropriate to ask teachers to assist with recruitment efforts.

Community Organizations as Referring Agents

Community organizations can be very helpful in recruiting participants for Homework Success. The directors of community organizations should be contacted by sending an introductory/recruitment letter. Homework Success information flyers should also be sent. Community organizations that could be considered for recruitment purposes include churches, home–school associations, neighborhood committees, and parent support/educational groups, such as Children and Adults with Attention Deficit Disorders (CHADD), although there may be many other organizations that clinicians will wish to contact. We suggest that clinicians maintain communication with the leaders of these organizations to promote integration within the overall community.

RECRUITING PARTICIPANTS FOR SCHOOL SETTINGS

The school is the ideal context within which to conduct Homework Success. The guidelines presented in the previous section pertaining to physicians and behavioral health professionals are applicable regardless of the intended setting of the program. This section describes special considerations for recruiting participants when the program is offered in school settings.

In-Service Training as a Recruitment Tool

When clinicians plan to conduct Homework Success in a school setting, teachers are clearly a very helpful source of referrals. However, teachers have been shown to vary greatly in their knowledge about ADHD and in their perceptions about the acceptability and utility of various interventions for this disorder (Power et al., 1995; Shapiro, DuPaul, Bradley, & Bailey, 1996). Because it has been shown that education about ADHD can change perceptions about the acceptability of interventions for this disorder (Liu et al., 1991), we recommend that in-service training be provided to teachers as a strategy to enlist their collaboration in recruiting families for Homework Success.

Packaged programs have been developed to assist with the in-service training of teachers regarding ADHD (e.g., see Fowler, 1992). We have found it especially useful to review facts and misconceptions about ADHD with teachers (see Karustis, Habboushe, & Power, 1997).

Following well-designed, well-organized in-service training about ADHD, teachers are in a much better position to make appropriate referrals to the Homework Success Program. Clinicians should inform teachers that families will be provided with support and assistance even in the event that they do not meet criteria for participation.

SCREENING POTENTIAL PARTICIPANTS

Once prospective participants have been referred, these families should be carefully screened. We recommend a multigate screening process that includes the following steps: (1) an initial telephone conversation with the family to identify type and level of concerns, (2) the completion of rating scales by parents and teachers, and (3) an interview with the family.

Selection Criteria

In order to participate in Homework Success, the referred child should be experiencing significant problems with homework. The clinician should also determine whether additional problems are present that may require further evaluation or alternative intervention programs. Furthermore, the parents must be ready and able to make a commitment to invest in the program in order for it to be successful. Specific screening criteria follow. (It should be noted that more stringent criteria may be required if a clinician is planning to conduct research using the program.)

The following primary questions should be addressed during the screening process:

1. Is the child experiencing significant homework problems?
2. Does the child have ADHD or problems related to ADHD that are contributing to homework impairments?
3. Are additional learning, emotional, and/or behavioral problems present that may require more individualized and intensive interventions in addition to or in lieu of Homework Success?
4. Are the parents prepared and able to commit to full participation in the program?

The screening process entails gathering information regarding the child's functioning in home and school settings. For this reason it is necessary to use a multiple-informant method. Information obtained from parents and teachers will in some cases indicate the need for more detailed assessment. Screening results that suggest significant cognitive and learning problems may require a comprehensive psychoeducational battery. A description of comprehensive psychoeducational assessment methods is beyond the scope of this manual. Such descriptions are presented in texts such as those by Anastasi and Urbina (1997), Barkley (1998), and Vance (1997). Screening results that indicate the presence of severe emotional disturbance, suicidality, and/or physically assaultive behaviors will require further assessment and possible interventions as an alternative to participation in Homework Success.

An issue of increasing concern and importance to clinicians that should be taken into account during any screening or assessment process is the appropriateness of rating scales for individuals of diverse backgrounds and cultures (Power, Eiraldi, Mercugliano, & Blum, 1998; Reid, 1995). Because the question of cultural sensitivity remains an open one, we suggest that clinicians interpret rating scale results carefully and augment these measures whenever possible with other methods, such as interviews, direct observations, and samples of children's work. The following is a description of recommended domains and instruments for screening.

Homework Problems

There are several methods for assessing problems with homework. For comprehensiveness and direct relevance to Homework Success, we recommend use of the Homework Performance Questionnaire (HPQ; Power, Karustis, Mercugliano, & Blum, 1999; see also Appendix B, this volume). The HPQ is a parent report measure that includes 12 homework-related behaviors (e.g., "Needs many reminders to begin homework") that are rated on a 4-point Likert scale. In addition, the HPQ includes sections in which parents indicate the duration of time spent on homework, percentage of homework completed, and quality of work for each subject area over the previous 2 weeks. This measure not only provides valuable information about the nature and severity of homework problems but also yields baseline data that will be useful for progress monitoring. It should be noted, however, that normative data on this measure have not yet been developed. The most appropriate way to use this measure is to compare child ratings to a criterion established by teachers and parents that reflects appropriate homework performance.

An alternative measure of homework issues is the Homework Problem Checklist (HPC; Anesko et al., 1987). The HPC is a 20-item parent report measure of problems with homework performance that employs a 4-point Likert scale. It has been normed for grades 2 through 4, with a total raw score of approximately 18 recommended as a cutoff for clinical significance (Kahle & Kelley, 1994). The HPC has been shown to be sensitive to intervention effects (Anesko et al., 1987) and thus can be used for the purposes of both screening and treatment evaluation. Because this measure has not been normed for the full range of students from grades 1 through 6, the norms should be used with caution.

If possible, clinicians should also collect information about children's actual homework performance. This can be done by asking parents to collect and submit all homework completed by their child for the previous week or two.

Symptoms of ADHD

As previously noted, an ADHD diagnosis is not necessary for participation in Homework Success. However, it is important for clinicians to identify whether the child has problems related to ADHD to determine whether the program may need to be modified slightly for certain families. Research has increasingly suggested that parent and teacher reports of behavior are perhaps the most crucial elements in determining a child's status regarding ADHD symptomatology (DuPaul & Stoner, 1994; Power, Andrews, et al., 1998).

Many norm-referenced scales for assessing ADHD are currently available. The ADHD Rating Scale–IV, Home and School Versions (ADHD-IV; DuPaul, Power, Anastopoulos, & Reid, 1998), are 18-item symptom checklists reflecting diagnostic criteria for ADHD as outlined in the fourth edition of the *Diagnostic and Statistical Manual of Mental Disorders* (American Psychiatric Association, 1994; see Table 2.1 in Chapter 2). The ADHD Rating Scale–IV is designed to assess inattention and hyperactivity–impulsivity in both home and school settings. For screening, the School Version can be completed by the child's current primary teacher, and the Home Version can be completed by the parent who is most involved in assisting the child with homework. Frequency of behaviors displayed over the past 6 months are rated on a 4-point Likert scale. Normative data for total scores, as well as for the Inattention and Hyperactivity–Impulsivity factors, are provided according to gender and age group.

Other widely used rating scales that can be employed for elementary school children include (1) the ADHD Symptom Checklist–4 (Gadow, 1997), (2) the Attention Deficit Disorders Evaluation Scale (ADDES; McCarney, 1996), (3) the ADD-H Comprehensive Teacher's Rating Scales (ACTeRS; Ullman, Sleator, Sprague, & MetriTech Staff, 1996), and (4) Conners' Rating Scales–Revised (Conners, 1997). For screening purposes, it is recommended that scores at or above the 90th percentile on the Inattention factor of either the parent or teacher rating ADHD scales be used as cutoffs for participation, as scores above this cutoff suggest the presence of some ADHD symptomatology in the child (Power, Andrews, et al., 1998).

Developmental and Learning Problems

A useful screening measure for identifying learning problems is the Academic Performance Questionnaire (APQ; Power, Karustis, et al., 1999; see also Appendix B, this volume). The APQ asks teachers to provide information regarding students' performance relative to that of classmates in major subject areas. Percent completion and accuracy rates are obtained in mathematics and written expression. Information regarding remedial services being provided to the child is also gathered, as are teacher ratings of the student's homework completion rates, homework quality, and homework difficulties. An alternate teacher report measure is the Academic Performance Rating Scale (DuPaul, Rapport, & Perriello, 1991; see also Appendix B, this volume), a 19-item, 5-point Likert scale measure that provides information pertaining to students' academic productivity and accuracy.

Before enrolling families into Homework Success, it is important for clinicians to know if children have significant impairments in cognitive, sensory, or neurological functioning that may have an impact on their homework performance. In many cases the nature and extent of these impairments have been assessed during evaluations conducted previously. During the screening process, parents should be asked if their child has received a psychological or psychoeducational evaluation over the past 3 years. If so, a copy of the evaluation report should be requested.

If the child has not been evaluated within the past 3 years and there are questions about cognitive and academic functioning, a brief cognitive and learning assessment should be conducted. Brief measures of intellectual functioning, such as the Wechsler Abbreviated Scale of Intelligence (WASI; Psychological Corporation, 1999) or the Kaufman Brief Intelligence Test (K-BIT; Kaufman & Kaufman, 1990), are easy to administer and may provide useful information. Brief measures of academic achievement that may be employed include the Kaufman Tests of Educational Achievement—Brief Form (K-TEA; Kaufman & Kaufman, 1985) and the Wechsler Individual Achievement Test Screener (Psychological Corporation, 1992). Indications of cognitive deficits, learning disabilities, or academic skills deficits should not be used to exclude children from Homework Success. Rather, this information may be helpful in addressing the child's learning needs and in modifying instructional programming.

Externalizing and Internalizing Problems

To assess children's emotional and behavioral problems, broadband behavior rating scales should also be included in the screening process and should be completed by both parents and teachers. Some of the more commonly used and well-normed scales are the Behavior Assessment System for Children (Reynolds & Kamphaus, 1992), the Child Behavior Checklist and Teacher Report Form (Achenbach, 1991a, b), and the Devereux Scales of Mental Disorders (Naglieri, LeBuffe, & Pfeiffer, 1994). Clinicians should pay particular attention to subscales pertaining to conduct problems and internalizing symptomatology. The presence of externalizing problems, such as noncompliance and defiance, is very common among children with ADHD (Biederman, Newcorn, & Sprich, 1991) and should not be used to exclude referred children from the group. However, screening results suggesting possible conduct disorder or physically assaultive behaviors in general should exclude a child from Homework Success. Likewise, symptoms of anxiety and depression that are highly elevated may be indicators of the need for alternate interventions, with possible suicidality requiring immediate attention by the clinician and family. On the other hand, elevated anxiety or depression scores on behavior rating scales are common among children with ADHD and should not automatically be used to exclude children from Homework Success.

Family Stress

Homework Success can provide a supportive context in which parents can discuss the stressors and conflicts they experience in their families. However, some parents may be coping with significant stress in their lives and may be in need of further evaluation and treatment. Parents coping with significant problems may not be able to commit and be responsive to Homework Success. To understand family factors that may have an impact on a family's ability to respond to the program, we recommend that clinicians schedule a conference with the parents to conduct an interview (see Chapter 6). During the interview the clinician can explore whether personal or family problems may interfere with success in treatment. For example, the clinician can learn whether physical health, mental health, marital problems, or financial issues may be impediments to intervention. Indications of physical, sexual, or emotional abuse should be explored to determine if a further assessment of these problems is indicated. The clinician needs to be sensitive in eliciting information regarding the parents' own functioning during the screening process, given that the primary focus of Homework Success is on helping the child, not the parents. In situations in which the parents are coping with significant stress, it may be wise to suspend involvement in Homework Success and develop an alternative intervention plan.

Readiness for Change

If a parent is not prepared to commit to Homework Success or does not believe that such a group can be helpful to the family, it is unlikely that consistent attendance, adherence to program strategies, and overall improvements in functioning will occur.

To assess readiness for change, the continuous-measure form of the Stages of Change Scale (McConnaughy, DiClemente, Prochaska, & Velicer, 1989; Prochaska et al., 1992) was developed based on the work of Prochaska and colleagues. This measure yields separate scores for each of the five stages of the model (Prochaska & DiClemente, 1992). As an alternative, Table 3.1 presents a series of questions, based on Prochaska's model, that can be useful to clinicians in assessing a family's readiness for change. Responses to these questions will provide the clinician with a sense of whether or not the parents are prepared for and able to commit to participation in Homework Success. Individuals who appear to be primarily at the preparation or action phases are appropriate for enrollment in Homework Success. An example of a response from a parent at the preparation stage is, "I have been thinking about getting help for my child and I am now ready to participate in a program to help my child." An individual at the action stage will have taken some actions recently, such as collaborating with the teacher to modify the homework assignment book and applying consequences, such as removal of the privilege of watching television, if assignments are not completed.

Families at the precontemplation stage rarely are referred to the program; these parents have not yet determined that their child has a problem with homework and needs help. Many referred families, however, are at the contemplation stage. These parents know that their child has a problem, but they are not sure what to do about it or whether they need to commit their time and energy to solve the problem. These families should not be enrolled in Homework Success until they have decided that the program can help them and that they are ready to make the necessary commitment. When families are at the contemplation stage, clinicians should attempt to identify potential obstacles to their participation in the program. Further education and consultation will help parents to decide whether they are ready to engage in Homework Success at this time.

The ADHD Knowledge and Opinion Survey (AKOS; Bennett et al., 1996) may be

TABLE 3.1. Interview Questions for Determining Readiness for the Homework Success Program

1. Does your child have problems with homework?
2. If yes, what do you see as your child's problems with homework?
3. How severe do you think these problems are?
4. Do you believe that you and your child need help with homework?
5. If yes, what kind of help do you think you need?
6. Based on what you know about Homework Success, do you think this program can help you and your child?
7. If yes, are you ready to make a commitment to this program at this time?
8. What factors might make it difficult for your family to fully particpate in Homework Success at this time?

very useful in assessing parents' attitudes about intervention and factors that may preclude them from being ready for a program like Homework Success. This 42-item parent report measure (see Appendix B) is divided into two sections: a 17-item true–false scale assessing parents' knowledge about ADHD and a 26-item scale presented in a 6-point Likert format assessing parents' willingness to use medication and psychosocial interventions, as well as their perceptions about the feasibility of participating in treatment. The AKOS provides normative data on four subscales: ADHD Knowledge, Counseling Acceptability, Medication Acceptability, and Counseling Feasibility.

The Counseling Acceptability and Feasibility factors are particularly relevant in screening families for Homework Success. For example, a sample item from the Counseling Acceptability scale is "Family therapy would probably be helpful to us." A sample item from the Counseling Feasibility scale is "Our family should have no difficulty traveling to and from counseling sessions." A low score (e.g., 1 standard deviation below the mean) may suggest that a parent is not ready to commit to Homework Success and initially should receive an alternative method of support. A low score on Counseling Feasibility may indicate that it is not feasible for the family to participate in Homework Success at this time.

When the Homework Success Program Is Not Appropriate

As discussed, the Homework Success Program is not appropriate for all referred families. Clinicians should be prepared to discuss options and to refer families to alternative programs and providers when Homework Success is not indicated. Guidelines for addressing the needs of families who cannot be served through this program follow.

Mild Homework- or ADHD-Related Problems

In some cases, results of the screening process will indicate that homework difficulties are not sufficiently problematic to warrant involvement in the comprehensive Homework Success Program. In these cases, clinicians may offer the parents brief consultation to address the child's homework difficulties. The strategies outlined in Chapters 6 through 9 pertaining to establishing collaborative home–school relationships, establishing a homework routine, assessing the nature and function of homework problems, and using positive reinforcement for productive homework behavior may be particularly useful to clinicians during these consultation meetings. Alternately, it may be that a resource list provided to the parents will be sufficient (see Handout 17, Appendix D).

Comorbid Conditions

As indicated, in situations in which the child has significant cognitive or learning problems that have not yet been assessed, an evaluation by the school psychologist is generally indicated. The clinician and family will need to decide whether to initiate Homework Success while awaiting this evaluation or to defer enrollment in the program until a comprehensive educational plan has been developed. If the presence of conduct disorder or physically assaultive behaviors is suggested via screening, the clinician should meet with the family to advise them of the need for alternative evaluation and intervention services. In these cases, the parents are advised to obtain a psychiatric or psychological evaluation before being enrolled in Homework Success. Also, children with severe anxiety and depressive symptoms should have these issues assessed prior to enrollment in a group program such as Homework Success. Clinicians should refer these families to a psychiatrist or psychologist for further assessment and treatment. Typically, these children will require specialized interventions to address their internalizing symptoms before being enrolled in Homework Success.

Not Ready for Change

In some cases a family will meet the inclusionary criteria given here, yet indications are that the parents are not yet prepared to benefit from a group program such as Homework Success. For example, parents may indicate that they are unsure what type of intervention their child needs for homework problems or that they are reluctant to commit to a seven-session group intervention. The clinician in these situations could provide parents with a list of resources, including readings and local self-help organizations. Parents should be encouraged to contact the clinician if they wish to participate in Homework Success in the future.

Feasibility Problems

A number of barriers to participation were discussed earlier in this chapter. Whenever possible, the clinician should help families to address feasibility problems. These problems include transportation, scheduling, sibling care, and financial barriers. When Homework Success is conducted in school or community settings, transportation barriers may be minimized. Likewise, sibling care arrangements may be easier to address in a community setting, and implementation of the program in a school setting will in many cases alleviate financial concerns regarding participation. Depending on the population served, scheduling of sessions will be more appropriate either during the day or evening hours. When feasibility barriers cannot be overcome, the clinician should meet with the family to discuss service options. Options may include referral to a publicly funded behavioral health clinic; a private provider who is in a network with the family's health insurance plan; or a school professional, such as a counselor or school psychologist.

## CHAPTER 4

Assessing Intervention Integrity and Evaluating Outcomes

SHEEBA DANIEL-CROTTY, DINA F. HABBOUSHE,
JAMES L. KARUSTIS, AND THOMAS J. POWER

For Homework Success to be effective, the key elements of the intervention program must be implemented as specified. In other words, the intervention strategies must be applied with integrity. In a family–school intervention program such as this, treatment integrity refers to the extent to which clinicians follow guidelines in providing the program and the extent to which parents and teachers participate in the program and implement recommended procedures. Another critical component of a successful intervention program is the comprehensive evaluation of outcomes. Outcome evaluation consists of formative methods to assess ongoing progress in meeting program objectives, as well as summative methods to determine the effects at the conclusion of the formal program and at various follow-up points.

This chapter presents procedures for assessing intervention integrity, as well as methods to monitor progress and evaluate summative program outcomes. An emphasis is placed on using multiple methods and multiple informants to comprehensively assess outcome. Further, methods to evaluate parents' and children's perceptions of the acceptability and reasonableness of the components of the program are described to provide an assessment of social validity.

MONITORING INTERVENTION INTEGRITY

An important step in determining whether Homework Success is having its intended effect is to carefully monitor the extent to which this structured, standardized program is being implemented by clinicians as intended. To assist with the monitoring of intervention integrity, checklists for each session have been developed (see Appendix C). Each checklist includes items pertaining to the content and process of sessions, as well as items referring to activities that are to be completed between sessions, such as telephone contact with teachers or parents.

The content section of the integrity checklists specifies each task that clinicians are expected to address during each session. The process section of the checklists specifies tasks that have been demonstrated to promote effective group process, such as ensuring participation of all group members and being responsive to participants' concerns (Schoenholtz-Read, 1994).

Checklists have been used in a variety of ways to improve and maintain the integrity of intervention programs (Ehrhardt et al., 1996). First, clinicians can use the checklists as a guide during sessions to prompt them to follow the tasks of the Homework Success Program. Clinicians are encouraged to self-monitor the integrity with which they are following the program by checking off tasks as they accomplish them. Second, the checklists can be completed by a supervisor, colleague, or research coordinator, and this information can be used to provide external feedback to the clinician regarding intervention integrity. Further, after videotaping training sessions, clinicians can observe the videos and use these checklists as a self-evaluation tool to improve and maintain the integrity of their intervention work.

The integrity of Homework Success interventions also depends on consistent application of program procedures by the family and teachers. For the program to be successful, family members need to attend the sessions, participate actively in the sessions, perform homework assignments, and complete outcome measures. Also, teachers need to check homework assignment books, negotiate with parents about realistic expectations for work completion, evaluate homework promptly, and complete outcome measures periodically. In implementing this program, clinicians are encouraged to keep weekly records regarding (1) parent and child attendance at sessions, (2) completion of homework assignments by parents, (3) level of participation of parents in training sessions, (4) checking and initialing of homework assignment books by teachers, (5) teacher willingness to negotiate with parents about expectations for work completion, and (6) completion of outcome measures by parents and teachers. To assist the clinician in checking integrity, parents are to submit homework assignments and data on outcome measures on a weekly basis. Also, parents are encouraged to bring the child's homework assignment book to sessions each weekly. We urge clinicians to rate each parent's level of participation at the conclusion of each group session. Further, it is useful to rate on an ongoing basis each teacher's willingness to collaborate with parents about recording homework assignments and setting expectations for homework performance.

EVALUATING INTERVENTION OUTCOME

To examine the effectiveness of Homework Success, the use of a multimethod, multiinformant battery of measures is recommended. Outcome measures should include methods that will facilitate ongoing progress monitoring, as well as comprehensive, summative evaluation. The program is designed to have positive effects on various domains of child and family functioning, including homework productivity, accuracy, and efficiency; academic functioning in the classroom; and family functioning. Therefore, comprehensive outcome evaluation for the program must involve one or more methods to assess each of these domains. Also, it is critical that a successful intervention program be socially valid—that is, goals, treatment procedures, and expected outcomes must be viewed as acceptable and reasonable by the consumers of the program (Kazdin, 1980; Schwartz & Baer, 1991). The following sections provide the rationale for evaluating each of the domains indicated and a description of recommended measures to assess each domain.

MEASURES OF HOMEWORK PRODUCTIVITY, ACCURACY, AND EFFICIENCY

An obvious goal of Homework Success is to improve homework performance. We expect that this program will improve the student's organizational skills, including completing the homework assignment book, transporting the assignment book and the appropriate classroom materials from school to home, having materials ready to complete homework, and starting homework on time at the assigned location. We expect that students will increase their attention to homework tasks, resulting in improvements in rates of homework completion. Also, we expect that children will become more accurate and careful in performing assignments. A further objective of the program is to enable children to work more efficiently, which for many children means a reduction in the amount of time spent on homework.

Homework Performance Questionnaire (HPQ)

The HPQ (Power, Karustis, et al., 1999; see also Appendix B, this volume) was designed to assess various aspects of homework performance, including preparedness for work, behavior during homework, rate of work completion, rate of work accuracy, and time spent on homework. Parents are requested to rate each of 12 homework difficulties on a scale from (*never a problem*) to 3 (*very often a problem*). Also, parents are asked to estimate the percentage of homework completed and the quality of homework in the areas of math, reading, and language arts over the previous 2 weeks. In addition, parents are requested to estimate the average daily time that their child has spent doing homework in math, reading, and language arts over the previous 2 weeks.

Parent-Reported Logs

Parents are asked to record homework accuracy, completion, and duration on a Daily Homework Log during the course of the program (Appendix B). On a recording sheet, parents are asked to document the number of problems assigned, completed, and correct for each written homework assignment. In addition, parents are to record the amount of time spent on each assignment and total time spent on homework each day. Completion rates are calculated by dividing the number of problems completed by the number of problems assigned and then multiplying by 100. Accuracy rates are calculated by dividing the number of problems correct by the number of problems completed and then multiplying by 100. Another index that has been demonstrated to be useful in evaluating intervention outcomes is the academic efficiency ratio, which reflects the number of problems correct divided by the number of problems assigned multiplied by 100 (Rapport et al., 1988).

Samples of Homework

A more objective source of information about homework performance is the actual homework that is completed by children. There are essentially two methods by which to collect samples of homework. One way is to ask teachers to collect and store the homework that children submit to them. Clinicians can request this information on a regular basis, score it, and return it to the teacher. Alternatively, teachers can return the homework to parents, who in turn can collect and store it. Periodically, parents can submit this information to clinicians for scoring. Generally, we have found that collecting homework samples directly from teachers is the most reliable method. Samples of homework can be scored for rates of completion, accuracy, and academic efficiency in a manner similar to that described for the parent-reported logs.

Teacher Logs of Homework Performance

Most teachers keep a log of homework completion, and some keep a more detailed record of accuracy. Although these data may vary depending on the level of detail of the teacher's records, they can be very useful in program evaluation. Because teacher logs represent data that already exist, additional effort on the teacher's part is not required to obtain this information. Also, these data are relatively free of contamination, in that the individuals collecting and recording the data (teachers) are different from the primary agents of the intervention (parents and children).

Goal-Setting Tool

The Goal-Setting Tool (Appendix D), which is described in detail in Chapter 10, is a worksheet that can be very helpful to families in managing time, setting goals, evaluating performance, and determining consequences for homework performance. On this worksheet the parents and child record data on a daily basis during and after the completion of each homework assignment. For example, the parents and child record data pertaining to (1) goals for work completion, accuracy, and duration; (2) actual number of items completed and performed accurately; (3) whether goals for completion and accuracy have been attained; and (4) points earned for work completion and accuracy that can be used in a token economy system. This worksheet yields a wealth of data that can be very helpful in evaluating the outcomes of the program. However, because this technique is not introduced until the fourth session of the program, it may be more useful in evaluating the efficacy of interventions introduced later in the session and the long-term effects of the program, as opposed to evaluating changes in performance from baseline to posttreatment.

MEASURES OF ACADEMIC FUNCTIONING

Although Homework Success does not directly target academic performance in the classroom, it is expected that this program will have some effects on student achievement in school. Because Homework Success should enable the child to attain better grades for homework performance and to be better prepared for class, it is anticipated that the quality of schoolwork should improve. Many parents and teachers expect that improvements in study habits during homework will generalize to work habits in the classroom. Although this is a desired outcome, many children, particularly those with ADHD, demonstrate significant problems generalizing behavior change from one setting to another (Barkley, 1998). For this reason, it is very important that teachers employ strategies in the classroom that are very similar to those used in Homework Success to improve academic performance in the classroom. The following measures are useful in assessing the effects of Homework Success on school performance:

Academic Performance Rating Scale (APRS)

The APRS (DuPaul et al., 1991; see also Appendix B, this volume) is a 19-item, teacher-rated questionnaire that assesses academic performance. Teachers are asked to estimate a student's rate of work completion and accuracy in the areas of math and language arts. Also, teachers rate the child's ability to pay attention, follow instructions, and learn in the classroom environment. The APRS yields scores on three factors: Academic Productivity, Academic Success, and Impulse Control. The psychometric properties of this measure have been carefully evaluated and have been demonstrated to be adequate (DuPaul et al., 1991). Because this instrument is brief and can be completed in less than 5 minutes, it is highly suitable for repeated measurement and progress monitoring.

Samples of Classwork

Student performance on work assigned in class is very easy to collect and score and is a valuable source of data about academic functioning. Classwork, like homework, can be scored for rates of work completion, accuracy, and efficiency.

Teacher Logs of Academic Performance

All teachers keep records of student performance on classwork assignments, tests, and quizzes. This information can be very useful in assessing the effects of Homework Success on academic performance in class. Because this information is kept routinely by the teacher, it requires very little effort to obtain these data. Many teachers are willing to make copies of these logs from their record book periodically so that this information can be used for progress monitoring.

MEASURES OF FAMILY FUNCTIONING

The Homework Success Program is designed to improve family relationships and to reduce parent-child conflict that often arises during homework. It is expected that establishing a homework routine, setting realistic goals for homework, reinforcing responsible homework behavior, and strategically using punishment will lead to a reduction in the number of arguments and negative interactions between the parent and child, and result in improvements in this relationship. Numerous measures are available to assess the impact of Homework Success on family functioning. We have found that the following rating forms are particularly useful in assessing changes in parent–child relationships and parenting stress.

Conflict Behavior Questionnaire (CBQ), Parent and Child Versions— Short Forms

The CBQ Short Forms (Robin & Foster, 1989; see also Appendix B, this volume) have been designed to assess perceived communication and conflict between parents and children aged 10 through 19, although we have found it to be useful with children as young as 8 years of age. Both the parent and child versions of the CBQ Short Forms consist of 20 true–false items. The items contained on these short forms are the items from the original CBQ that demonstrated the highest correlation with full-scale scores and that best differentiated distressed from nondistressed parent–child dyads (Robin & Foster, 1989). Because these scales are brief and easy to complete, they are well suited for repeated use as outcome measures.

Parenting Stress Index (PSI)—Short Form

The PSI–Short Form (Abidin, 1995) is a very useful measure of parent-reported stress associated with parenting and family variables (e.g., health, marital, and economic concerns), as well as child variables (e.g., activity level and moodiness of the child). The PSI–Short Form is a 36-item questionnaire that uses a 5-point Likert-type format. This measure yields indices of stress related to parent variables and child variables, as well as a total stress score. Psychometric properties, including internal consistency, test–retest reliability, and discriminant validity have been demonstrated to be adequate (Abidin, 1995). Although the PSI–Short Form is recommended as a measure of outcome, we view this scale as an adjunctive measure to be used if the clinician is particularly interested in assessing the impact of the program on parenting stress.

EVALUATING INTERVENTION ACCEPTABILITY AND CONSUMER SATISFACTION

Another important aspect of program evaluation is the continuous assessment of intervention acceptability. Acceptability has been defined as perceptions by consumers that interventions are appropriate, fair, and reasonable for the clients and problems for which they are being used (Kazdin, 1980). Interventions that are acceptable to parents, teachers, and children are more likely to be implemented and applied with integrity than treatments that are viewed as unreasonable or inappropriate in some way. Therefore, it is very important that clinicians understand at the outset how their clients perceive the interventions that will be used and collaborate with families and school professionals to design strategies that are perceived to be potentially effective and reasonable. In addition, because the acceptability of interventions can change during the course of treatment, it is essential that clinicians periodically reassess perceptions about the reasonableness of intervention approaches (Reimers, Wacker, Cooper, & DeRaad, 1992). By evaluating treatment acceptability on an ongoing basis, group leaders are better able to respond to each family's changing needs throughout the program.

Clinicians should also request that parents provide a formal evaluation scale of Homework Success at the end of the program. We have developed a program evaluation that is particularly suited to assessing parent satisfaction with the Homework Success Program. The following measures of intervention acceptability and consumer satisfaction are recommended.

Homework Success Evaluation Inventory (HSEI)

The HSEI (Appendix B) is a seven-item rating scale designed to assess parents' views about the fairness, reasonableness, and potential helpfulness of Homework Success. Parents are asked to rate each item on a 6-point Likert scale ranging from 1 (*strongly disagree*) to 6 (*strongly agree*). The scale is intentionally brief so that it is feasible to use on a repeated basis. Research has demonstrated that brief acceptability measures such as this have strong psychometric properties and can be very useful in assessing social validity (Kelley, Heffer, Gresham, & Elliott, 1989; Power et al., 1995).

Children's Intervention Rating Profile (CIRP)

The CIRP (Witt & Elliot, 1985; see also Appendix E, this volume) is a seven-item questionnaire used to assess children's perceptions of treatment acceptability. The CIRP is very commonly used in research and practice to assess children's views about the social appropriateness of various approaches to intervention. We have adapted the scale slightly to make it appropriate for use with this program.

Homework Success Program Evaluation Scale

This questionnaire was designed to assess parent satisfaction with the Homework Success Program (Appendix B). It consists of 16 items rated on a 5-point Likert scale from

1 (*not helpful*) to 5 (*extremely helpful*). Parents are asked to evaluate each of the major topics included in the program. They are also asked to indicate their satisfaction with the organization of the group and the responsiveness of the group leader. The questionnaire also contains two open-ended items asking parents to comment on aspects of the program that were most helpful and to make suggestions for improving the program in the future. Although this inventory was developed specifically for Homework Success, some clinicians may prefer to develop their own measure or to use questionnaires developed by other researchers, such as the Parent Consumer Satisfaction Questionnaire (Forehand & McMahon, 1981).

TIMETABLE FOR DATA COLLECTION

Collecting data using multiple methods and multiple informants on an ongoing basis is essential for progress monitoring and outcome assessment. Table 4.1 provides a suggested timetable for collecting data pertaining to the measures described in this chapter. In the description of each program session, group leaders are prompted to collect data pertaining to each of these measures.

TABLE 4.1. Recommended Timetable for Collecting Outcome Data

Measure	Parent meeting	Home–school meeting	Session 1	Session 2	Session 3	Session 4	Session 5	Session 6	Session 7
HPQ	×			×		×		×	×
Daily logs			×	×	×	×	×	×	×
Work samples	×			×		×		×	×
Teacher records		×		×		×		×	×
APRS		×		×		×		×	×
CBQ			×						×
HSEI	×			×		×		×	×

Note. HPQ, Homework Performance Questionnaire; APRS, Academic Performance Rating Scale; CBQ, Conflict Behavior Questionnaire—Parent and Child Forms; HSEI, Homework Success Evaluation Inventory.

CHAPTER 5

Setting Up the Program: Practical Considerations

To be effective, Homework Success must be provided in a context that is comfortable and accessible to families and that is conducive to collaboration and problem solving. As described in the Preface, Homework Success can be provided either in a group format or to one family at a time. This chapter focuses primarily on organizational and process-related issues that must be considered in implementing Homework Success in a group format, although some of the issues discussed also apply when the program is offered on an individualized basis. In this chapter, we provide guidelines for identifying appropriate clinicians, determining the optimal setting, organizing the group, and managing time effectively. In addition, suggestions for addressing the challenges presented by diverse participants are discussed.

IDENTIFYING APPROPRIATE CLINICIANS

This program should be conducted by professionals with advanced training in child development, psychopathology, behavioral principles, family systems theory, and home–school collaboration. For clinicians who will be implementing Homework Success in a group format, extensive knowledge about group counseling is also important. Clinicians meeting these criteria have training in a variety of disciplines, including clinical and school psychology, child psychiatry, social work, counseling, and pediatric nursing.

DETERMINING THE SETTING

In many cases the clinician will decide to conduct Homework Success in an outpatient clinic. Such settings have an advantage over school and community settings in allowing the clinician to more readily safeguard confidentiality. There is also a potential benefit to the clinician in having quicker access to materials and equipment from the clinic.

On the other hand, there are many potential benefits to conducting Homework Success in school and community settings. First, parents may be reluctant to attend a program at a clinic perceived as a center for treating "problem families." A school or community center is likely to be a familiar setting in which families are more comfortable than in an outpatient clinic. Second, implementing the program within schools may increase its accessibility (Power et al., 1994). Third, situating the program in a school facilitates greater involvement by the teacher. Given the frequent and often severe home–school communication problems reported by teachers pertaining to homework (Buck et al., 1996; Jayanthi, Sawyer, Nelson, Bursuck, & Epstein, 1995), conducting Homework Success in a school affords frequent opportunities for home–school collaboration to resolve these difficulties. Clinicians are well situated to attend home–school meetings to promote collaboration and problem solving and to reduce the stress that parents often experience at meetings with numerous professionals. Fourth, conducting the program in a school location opens avenues of communication between the clinician and teachers, thereby facilitating follow-up consultation. A further advantage of school-based programming is the accessibility of valuable, naturalistic data that are extremely useful in progress monitoring and outcome assessment (Power et al., 1994).

Clinicians may also wish to conduct Homework Success in a community setting. Conducting group programs such as Homework Success in community settings has been found to reduce barriers to family involvement in behavioral health services (Cunningham et al., 1995). Community settings, such as libraries, churches, and neighborhood centers, may be more familiar and accessible to families than are schools. Community settings are often perceived by families as stable and safe environments in which families feel understood and accepted (Ho, 1997). Many community settings also have an advantage in that they are frequently open in the evenings or on weekends. Curran (1989) reported that consumers of mental health services generally preferred a church locale to a school, hospital, or behavioral health facility. Community centers, libraries, and recreation centers were preferred next and were perceived as relatively welcoming and nonthreatening. If a church is used, clinicians are advised to obtain sponsorship from several churches to avoid the possible misperception that a particular doctrinal approach to parenting is being endorsed (Curran, 1989).

INVOLVING MULTIPLE CAREGIVERS

Whenever possible, we strongly recommend that all caregivers who are involved or who could become involved in assisting the child with homework be enlisted in the program. The involvement of multiple caregivers can improve the consistency with which homework strategies are applied, which is likely to result in better homework performance. In two-parent families, every effort should be made to involve both parents. For single-parent families, grandparents or friends are often involved in a child's homework, so they should be invited to attend sessions. Similarly, in situations in which the child is not living with a parent or grandparent, it is often appropriate to include multiple caregivers.

DECIDING WHETHER TO CONDUCT THE CHILD GROUP

Once a location has been determined, the group leader must ascertain whether the setting lends itself to conducting the concurrent child group and whether there are sufficient resources to do so. It is strongly recommended that the child group be conducted with the parent group whenever possible. Necessary resources for the child group include an individual with sufficient training to conduct the child group, at least one assistant, and adequate rooms and materials for both the parent and child groups. The child-group leader should be a professional with training and experience similar to those of the parent-group leader. Alternately, the child-group leader may be a graduate student who is working under the supervision of an experienced provider. See Chapter 14 for guidelines about conducting the child group and coordinating the parent and child groups.

ENSURING CONFIDENTIALITY

The clinician must ensure that each family's rights to privacy are protected. Clinic settings provide natural safeguards to confidentiality. If the program is held in a school or community setting, however, the clinician must provide explicit directions to participants to maintain confidentiality. For example, a general rule of Homework Success is that parents are not allowed to reveal any information shared by a participant in the group with any individual outside the group. Closed-door sessions and the use of sound screens are recommended. When the parents are asked to sign a release form to enable the clinician to speak with the teacher, the form must specify exactly what types of information can be discussed.

SETTING THE TIME FRAME

Each Homework Success session can be conducted in 90 minutes. Sessions should be held at a time that is mutually convenient for the participants and group leaders. Every effort should be made to minimize the amount of time parents need to spend outside the home, particularly during periods when the child should be doing homework. For parents who work outside the home, evening or weekend sessions may be optimal.

TAKING CARE OF SIBLINGS

One barrier to participation often reported by parents is the inability to obtain child-care services on a weekly basis. If a child group is being conducted, siblings of the referred child who are in grades 1 through 6 may also participate. If the child group is not being conducted, or if there are siblings in need of supervision who are not in elementary school, the group leader should consider providing child-care services.

SETTING UP THE ROOM

It is recommended that the group leader arrange seats in order to maximize eye contact among participants. If there is one door to the room, it should be in the back to minimize disruptions from any late arrivals. A blackboard or dry-erase board should be available during each session. The group leader may also wish to use videotaping equipment, if it is available, for use in modeling strategies and program techniques. Parents should be seated around a table so that they have a surface on which to place materials and take notes.

ARRANGING BREAKS

We recommend that clinicians plan for a brief (approximately 10-minute) break at the midpoint of each session. To model the importance of being prompt and efficient, it is important that sessions begin and conclude at the stated times. Likewise, clinicians should strive to be on time with the beginning and ending of breaks. It can be particularly difficult to reconvene from breaks. Informing the participants a minute or so before a break is over typically helps this process. Also, we recommend that group leaders provide refreshments for participants.

ATTENDING TO GROUP PROCESS

Throughout the program, but especially in the first session, emphasis is placed on the core factors that have been found to be related to behavior change in group interventions—namely, instilling hope, promoting a sense of a common mission, and imparting ground rules about group intervention to participants (Vinogradov & Yalom, 1989). In addition to ensuring that the instructional content of sessions is delivered, the group leader must work to facilitate group process (see Bernard & MacKenzie, 1994). It is essential that each parent participate during the sessions, that no one parent or clique of parents dominate, and that parental questions and individual family needs are addressed. The integrity checklists that are provided for each session (see Appendix C) include items to ensure that elements of group process are addressed. These elements are often difficult to maintain, given the variety of personalities and needs of participants. The diversity of participants can serve as a real strength for the group if the group leader is active in engaging each participant and in promoting interaction among participants. The group leader should be prepared to deal effectively and professionally with each parent in the interests of the entire group. The following discussion, although a generalization, should assist group leaders in addressing the challenges presented by the wide range of personalities served by this program (see also Curran, 1989).

The Passive Parent

Occasionally the group leader will encounter a parent who defers to other participants and who rarely, if ever, volunteers experiences and opinions. The group leader should encourage the passive parent to talk by directing specific questions to her or him and by praising attempts at participation. At several points during each session, the group leader should go around the room to obtain feedback from each participant. In some instances the passive parent will be one member of a couple, with the other member doing most or all of the participating. The group leader should make efforts to elicit participation from both partners.

The Assisting Parent

Some groups will include a participant who is extremely free in giving advice to other parents, behavior that may or may not be consistent with the principles and techniques presented by the group leader. It is important not to inhibit the assisting parent's enthusiasm. However, when appropriate, the group leader must make clear any substantial deviations from the Homework Success curriculum. Firm but polite ways in which to redirect the conversation include, "There are any number of ways we could deal with that, but right now let's stick to the program," and "What we've learned from running Homework Success over the years is that. . . . " The group leader may also wish to give a special responsibility to the assisting parent, such as telling the leader when it is time for a break or reconvening the group. We have found that this intervention is often sufficient to reduce excessive or inappropriate assisting.

The Dominating Parent

A frequent occurrence in groups is the parent who is so eager to participate and to get as much as possible from the program that he or she dominates discussions. It is recommended that the group leader praise appropriate participation from the dominating person while ensuring that each participant gets an opportunity to speak. It may be helpful to mention at the outset of the program that the leader will make sure that each person has an opportunity to participate and that a 2-minute limit on making comments will be used. In this manner no person should feel singled out or reprimanded, and the group leader is more able to maintain control over the pace of the session. For more extreme cases, the group leader may need to interrupt the dominating parent and say, "I just want to make sure that everybody is heard. Does anyone else want to say anything about this point?"

The Perfect Parent

Occasionally a parent who presents as needing help during the screening process will convey the impression of being "nearly perfect" as a parent during the group. This situation occurs more frequently when a couple attends the sessions. If a perfect parent emerges in the group, it is recommended that the group leader intervene by saying something like, "It sounds like you've tried many of the things we're presenting here—that's good. Now what sort of assistance would you like to obtain in this program?"

The Whining Parent

There is a fine line between expressing one's problems and whining. The whining parent is often not apparent until a session or two has passed, because during the initial phases of Homework Success the group leader will be actively encouraging participants to verbalize their experiences and problems. However, over time the whining parent will stand out by verbalizing the same problems without necessarily following through on the between-session assignments or without making a shift from a blaming perspective to an action-oriented stance. It is recommended that the group leader attempt to keep the whining parent on track by emphasizing the requirement of completing between-session assignments. The group leader should also elicit from the whining parent specific actions that will be taken between sessions and provide support in troubleshooting potential obstacles that may preclude follow through on these tasks.

The "Yes, But . . . " Parent

Occasionally the group leader will encounter a parent who responds to the presentation of an intervention strategy or between-session assignment with "Yes, but. . . . " This can take the form of excuses for noncompliance with assignments or of various reasons why a particular strategy has not or will not be effective. Such people can be frustrating to the group leader and disheartening to the other participants unless dealt with effectively. Particularly for these parents, clinicians should emphasize the importance of taking responsibility for following through on assignments. For example, the group leader may say, "Each family will have to tailor these ideas to fit their own particular needs. In what way can you do this?" Alternately the group leader might say, "Let's focus for a minute on why you don't think this will work in your family," and subsequently engage the person in a troubleshooting discussion.

The Rambling Parent

Parents of children with ADHD are more likely to have ADHD themselves than are parents of children without ADHD (Barkley, 1998). Whether or not ADHD has been diagnosed in a parent participant, the program will occasionally include a parent who has trouble stating ideas clearly and succinctly. The group leader may need to periodically interrupt such a person to either summarize (e.g., "What I hear you saying is that. . . . ") or to provide clarification to the person (e.g., "So are you saying that . . . ?"). As with the dominating parent, the group leader may also need to interrupt in order to move the session along and to ensure that all participants are heard.

The Stubborn Parent

Rarely do adults kick and scream in a manner similar to their children. Adult temper tantrums tend to be much more sophisticated, but what they have in common with children's tantrums is the unspoken premise, "Things shouldn't be this way!" The stubborn parent often makes statements such as, "I shouldn't have to praise my child for what she should already be doing anyway!" and "We didn't have any of this ADHD stuff when I was a kid." We have found that the most effective way of assisting the stubborn parent is to agree that things should not be this way but that we must begin with the way matters are, not with where we would like them to be.

The Theorizing Parent

The theorizing parent is one who spends an inordinate amount of time speculating about why children behave a certain way or how his or her parenting has evolved. If there is a theorizing parent in the group, there is a risk of other participants becoming disengaged or dropping out of the program. The group leader must directly state to the theorizing parent that Homework Success is an action-oriented program and that he or she is welcome to discuss theories with interested parties at the break or the conclusion of the session.

The Squabbling Couple

Sometimes it is difficult for a couple to shift from a blaming perspective to one that is solution oriented. In such instances the group leader is advised to emphasize the commonality of problems experienced by participants and should stress that "we're all in this together." Couples who persist in blaming one another should be asked to continue their particular discussion at the conclusion of the group. If indicated, the group leader can make himself or herself available for a couples session to work on the conflict.

The Overachieving Parent

This refers to the parent whose family appears to be making substantial gains almost from the start of the program. As such, it would be inappropriate to consider the overachieving parent a problem. However, because families vary to a great extent in the pace of their progress over the course of Homework Success, the group leader must be sure to remind participants that each family will make progress at different rates. For those participants who may be inclined to feel intimidated or disheartened by the overachieving parent, the group leader should stress the progress that has been made relative to their own baseline.

ADDRESSING NONCOMPLIANCE WITH PROGRAM REQUIREMENTS

Parents who have difficulty respecting confidentiality should be reminded about the centrality of this issue to the therapeutic process. In those rare cases in which a parent repeatedly violates principles of confidentiality, the group leader may need to encourage the person to suspend his or her involvement in the group. In some cases a person may frequently come late to sessions. Group leaders should remind participants about the importance of arriving on time for sessions. Likewise, if a participant is routinely late in returning from breaks, a reminder should be given. In all cases, the group leader should begin and end sessions and breaks at the stated times, regardless of whether or not the entire group is present.

There are also occasions on which parents do not or only partially comply with between-session assignments. When this occurs, the group leader should identify what the parents have completed and offer verbal praise. However, the group leader should also emphasize to parents that they cannot expect to derive significant benefits from Homework Success if they do not fully participate in the program. Because there are often significant obstacles to parental completion of assignments, the group leader should provide assistance in addressing the challenges. It is recommended that the group leader begin by making sure that the participants understand the directions for assignments. If time constraints are presented as barriers to adherence, the group leader can provide assistance in organizing time to increase the likelihood that between-session assignments will be completed. Chapter 9 provides additional guidelines for addressing nonadherence with between-session assignments.

ADDRESSING QUESTIONS ABOUT MEDICATION

Parents are asked to keep their child's medication status stable throughout the course of the program. Clinicians should encourage parents to inform them if a change in medication is anticipated. We recommend that group leaders meet with parents and confer with prescribing physicians to ascertain whether a change in medication or dosing is needed at this time. Of course, some children will require adjustments in medication during the program, and in these cases group leaders should not dissuade parents from making these adjustments. If there is a change in medication or dosing, clinicians should note when the adjustment was made, monitor the effects of the medication adjustment by using parent and teacher rating scales, and document these changes. Once medication status is stabilized, clinicians should reestablish the child's baseline level of functioning and monitor progress in relation to the original and the adjusted baseline levels.

CHAPTER 6

Initiating the Program

For Homework Success to be effective, it is critical to select families who are appropriate for this intervention, to prepare the families for the program, and to engage the parents and teachers in a collaborative consultation process. We strongly recommend that clinicians establish two meetings before initiating the parent-training component of the program. The first meeting is to be scheduled with the parents. The second meeting is to be scheduled at school with the parents and teachers. The following are specific guidelines for conducting each of these sessions.

PARENT CONFERENCE

> **GOALS**
>
> 1. Make sure the family meets program screening criteria.
> 2. Establish rapport and orient parents to the program.
> 3. Clarify program expectations.
> 4. Prepare for the parent–teacher meeting.
> 5. Complete baseline measures.

This meeting should be scheduled at the clinician's office at the convenience of the parents. Clinicians should allow at least 1 hour for this meeting and should encourage both parents to attend, when appropriate.

Goal 1: Make Sure the Family Meets Program Screening Criteria

As discussed in Chapter 3, it is essential to conduct a careful screening of the child and family before enrolling them in Homework Success. The screening contains four parts: (1) assessment of homework problems, (2) assessment of ADHD symptoms, (3) assessment of learning, emotional, and behavioral problems, and (4) assessment of the family's readiness for change. We encourage clinicians to obtain parent responses to the Homework Performance Questionnaire (HPQ); ADHD Rating Scale–IV; a multiaxial measure, such as the Child Behavior Checklist or Behavior Assessment System for Children (BASC), and the ADHD Knowledge and Opinion Scale (AKOS) prior to the parent conference. When appropriate, clinicians are advised to acquire records of previous psychological or learning evaluations. Also, clinicians should obtain teacher responses to the ADHD Rating Scale–IV, the Academic Performance Questionnaire (APQ), and the CBCL or BASC. Clinicians should score these scales and review parent and teacher responses before the meeting. During the conference they should review responses to these measures and ask the parents to clarify points that are unclear.

- Review responses to the HPQ to make sure the child is having significant homework problems. If the child's homework difficulties are minor, a one- or two-session consultation with a clinician may be more appropriate than the comprehensive Homework Success Program (see discussion in Chapter 3).
- Review parent and teacher responses to the ADHD Rating Scale–IV. It is not essential that the child have a definite diagnosis of ADHD in order for the family to be enrolled in the program. However, it is important that the child display many of the symptoms of ADHD, because the Homework Success strategies are designed for families coping with ADHD and many of the parents in the program will be discussing issues pertaining to ADHD, including diagnostic questions and medication concerns.
- Review teacher responses to the APQ. Identify learning problems that the child is experiencing. Make sure that the child's learning problems have been properly assessed and are being addressed by the school.
- Review parent and teacher responses to the BASC. Many of the families who are enrolled in Homework Success have children who display oppositional behavior and experience some level of anxiety and/or depression. If it is clear that the child displays moderate to severe behavior or emotional problems, then it may be more appropriate to refer the child and family for individualized therapy before enrolling them in Homework Success.
- Review parent responses to items on the AKOS. Also conduct a brief interview with the parents to identify the family's readiness for an intervention such as Homework Success (see Table 3.1 in Chapter 3). Chapter 3 provides guidelines for conducting this interview. Use the AKOS to identify potential obstacles to the family in becoming invested in the program. For example, identify problems with payment, family scheduling, child care, and transportation that might interfere with family participation. Make sure the family is ready to invest in Homework Success. If it is not feasible for the family to make a commitment to this program, provide them with appropriate alternatives.

Goal 2: Establish Rapport and Orient Parents to the Program

From the beginning, it is important to establish a relationship with the parents that is warm and trusting. Also, parents need to know (1) the goals of the program, (2) strategies that will be taught, (3) the importance of working collaboratively with the teacher, (4) procedures for evaluating progress and outcomes, (5) the importance of completing family homework assignments, (6) the schedule and time frame, (7) information about cost and potential for third-party reimbursement, and (8) information about transportation and parking. Further, clinicians need to explain whether a concurrent child group will be offered and, if so, how children will be involved in the program.

- Spend a few minutes establishing rapport with the parents.
- Distribute *Handout 1: Welcome to the Homework Success Program!* (Appendix D)
- Describe the goals of the program:

    1. Improving rates of homework completion and accuracy and improving the child's efficiency in completing homework.
    2. Improving the child's academic functioning.
    3. Improving the parent–child relationship.
    4. Reducing parent stress.

- Describe the strategies contained within Homework Success, including the following:

    1. Establishing a reliable way of reporting homework assignment.
    2. Establishing a homework routine.
    3. Giving instructions appropriately.
    4. Developing a system of positive reinforcement.
    5. Managing time and setting goals for homework.
    6. Using punishment successfully.
    7. Integrating and maintaining homework strategies.

- Describe to parents the important role of teachers and how teachers will be involved in the program. Tell them that a meeting with the teacher will be scheduled shortly to engage the teachers in the program. Also, tell the parent that teachers will be contacted later in the program to maintain effective home–school collaboration and to elicit the teachers' assistance with the strategies.
- Explain to parents the importance of monitoring progress and evaluating outcome to make sure the program is having its intended effects. Explain that the parents and teachers will complete measures pertaining to homework performance, academic functioning, family functioning, and parent and child attitudes about the appropriateness of the interventions.
- Emphasize to parents the importance of completing between-session assignments. Tell them that at the end of each session, parent homework assignments will be provided.
- Inform parents about scheduling issues. Indicate the date, time, and length of the program. Explain that the program will be offered in six sessions scheduled weekly. A follow-up meeting will be scheduled about 4 weeks after the sixth session and periodically after that, as indicated.

- Provide information about the cost of the program, methods of payment, and possibilities for obtaining third-party reimbursement.
- Inform parents about methods of transportation available to them. Also, let them know the arrangements for parking. We strongly recommend that arrangements be made to secure free parking or reduced fees for parking, particularly in cases in which the costs for the program are relatively high.
- Explain to parents how children will be involved in the intervention. If a concurrent child group will be offered, tell them to bring their child to the program each week. Explain to parents that the purpose of the child group is to introduce homework strategies so that the child understands the interventions and will be willing to cooperate with the parents and teachers in implementing them.

Goal 3: Clarify Program Expectations

Parents need to know what will be expected of them during the program so they can make the necessary arrangements and properly prepare themselves and their child.

- Stress that attendance at each session is very important. Parents should call when they cannot attend a session. Arrangements will be made to inform the parents about what they missed over the telephone or, if possible, right before the next session if they can arrive early.
- Urge both parents in a two-parent family to come to program sessions. Homework Success is likely to be most effective when both parents are involved in helping the child with homework. In single-parent families, the parent can be encouraged to bring a grandparent, family member, or friend to assist with the implementation of the strategies.
- Emphasize that homework assignments must be completed on time to master the strategies of Homework Success and to model responsible homework behavior for the child.
- Emphasize the importance of completing outcome measures at the assigned times to help with progress monitoring and outcome assessment.
- Explain the importance of stabilizing the medication status of the child during the program. Given that medication, particularly the stimulants, can have such marked effects on child behavior, explain to the parents that it will be difficult to assess the effects of Homework Success if medication status fluctuates throughout the course of the program. Urge parents to address any needed adjustments in medication before the start of the first parent-training session.

Goal 4: Prepare for the Parent–Teacher Meeting

Shortly after the parent conference, a parent–teacher meeting will be scheduled. Parents need to understand the role of the teacher in completing homework and the importance of home–school collaboration to improve homework performance. Also, parents need to understand the purpose and expected outcomes of the parent–teacher meeting.

• Explain the role of the teacher in completing homework assignments. Indicate that the teacher determines:

1. Type of homework assigned.
2. Amount of homework.
3. Method of informing students about assignments.
4. Method of assisting students in recording homework.
5. Method of evaluating homework.

• Explain the importance of home–school collaboration. Parents need to know from teachers how much homework will be assigned, how much time the child should spend on homework, what assistance the teacher will provide in recording assignments, and how homework will be evaluated. Teachers need to know from parents whether assignments are clearly recorded by the child, how much time is being spent doing homework, and what parents are doing to help the child complete homework accurately. When parents and teachers are working collaboratively, this information can be exchanged readily. When the relationship is not collaborative, parents and teachers do not get the information they need to help the child.

• Explain to parents the goals of the parent–teacher meeting (see the next section). Tell the parents that their role in the meeting includes the following steps:

1. Establish a cooperative relationship.
2. Praise the teacher in specific ways for helping the child.
3. Learn about their child's homework problems.
4. Learn about the types of homework assigned.
5. Find out how the teacher informs students about homework and how much assistance is provided in recording assignments.
6. Learn how much time the child should be spending on homework.
7. Learn about how the teacher evaluates the child's homework.
8. Describe the child's approach to homework.
9. Describe how much time it takes to do homework.
10. Describe the impact of homework on the family.
11. Ask the teacher to help the child in recording assignments, if needed.
12. Check to see if the teacher would allow the parents to place absolute limits on the amount of time spent on homework.
13. Ask the teacher to modify methods of evaluating homework if all work is not completed within the absolute time frame for homework.

Goal 5: Complete Baseline Measures

To monitor progress and evaluate outcomes, it is essential that parents complete outcome measures. The following measures should be completed:

• Parent-rated logs of homework completion, accuracy, and efficiency. Distribute log sheets (Appendix B) and explain to parents how to complete these forms. Ask parents to begin filling out the log sheets immediately and to do so on a daily basis throughout the program.

> • Parenting Stress Index—Short Form, if used. Ask parents to complete this scale during the parent conference.

> • Homework Success Evaluation Inventory. Ask parents to complete this form (Appendix B) during the conference. Tell parents to complete this scale based on their current understanding of the program as explained during the parent conference.

PARENT–TEACHER CONFERENCE

GOALS

1. Identify homework problems and resources.
2. Emphasize the importance of home–school collaboration.
3. Describe the Homework Success Program.
4. Enlist the teacher's assistance with homework.
5. Enlist the teacher's support in evaluating program outcomes.

This meeting should be scheduled in school at the convenience of the teacher and parents. At least 1 hour should be allotted for this conference.

Goal 1: Identify Homework Problems and Resources

Parents and teachers usually have no difficulty identifying homework difficulties, and this can be a useful way to get the meeting started and to help them become engaged with each other. It is important, however, to identify resources available in school and at home to instill hope and to assist with intervention planning.

> • Ask parents and teacher to identify homework problems. Request that they be specific and make a list of the stated problems.

> • Ask parents and teacher to identify homework resources. For example, schools often mandate the use of a homework assignment book, and some have homework hotlines available, that is, phone numbers parents and children can call to learn about homework assignments for a particular class. Also, the teacher may be accustomed to assigning a buddy to assist students in recording assignments. At home, both parents may be available to help the child, and the parents may be strict about not allowing the child to watch TV until homework has been completed. An additional resource is the parents' enrollment in Homework Success.

Goal 2: Emphasize the Importance of Home–School Collaboration

Problems with homework are often complicated to resolve and can have marked effects on academic performance and family functioning. Parents and teachers have complementary roles in addressing and overcoming homework problems. Parents and teachers need to understand that close collaboration is essential to improve homework performance.

- Explain how homework problems can affect academic performance by depriving the child of opportunities to practice and master skills and by lowering grades for homework that can lead to lower overall grades.
- Explain how homework problems can affect family functioning by contributing to frustration and anger in the child, stress in the parent, and parent–child conflict and by taking time away from other family issues, including time spent with other family members.
- Encourage the parents and teacher to identify together the roles each party has in assisting children with homework. For example, the teacher has a key role in determining the type and amount of homework assigned, how assignments are presented to children, and how homework is evaluated. Parents have a critical role in establishing the time and place for homework, in helping children to get started, to manage their time, and to stay on task and productive, and in determining the consequences of homework. Record on two lists the role of the teacher and the role of parents in assisting children with homework. This discussion will help to highlight the complementary roles of parents and teacher in homework and the importance of effective home–school collaboration.

Goal 3: Describe the Homework Success Program

Most teachers are very impressed when they learn about the commitment parents are making to help their child to do well in school by becoming involved in Homework Success. Often this will result in a renewed commitment on the part of the teacher to help the child.

- Describe for the teacher the goals of Homework Success, as outlined earlier in this chapter.
- Describe briefly for the teacher some of the strategies taught to parents during the program, as listed earlier in the chapter.

Goal 4: Enlist the Teacher's Assistance with Homework

At the outset of Homework Success, it is very important that the teacher provide the child with a basic level of support for homework. The child needs a method to record assignments and assistance to make sure assignments are recorded accurately and legibly. The parents need to know the absolute time limits for homework and how the teacher will evaluate work that is not completed beyond the absolute time limit.

- Ask the teacher to describe the method of instructing students about homework assignments. Ask him or her to describe the assistance that is available to ensure that assignments are recorded accurately and legibly. Ask the parents to describe their experiences at home understanding their child's communications regarding homework assignments. Facilitate a discussion between the parents and teacher to design a plan that will ensure that homework assignments are consistently recorded in a manner that is accurate and clear to parents.

- Ask the teacher to identify the maximum amount of time that children should be spending on homework. Ask the parents to describe the amount of time their child spends doing homework. Request that the parents and teacher define the absolute time limit for homework.

- Encourage parents to describe the consequences of applying the recommended absolute time limit for homework. Many parents fear that the child will not complete work, that work will not be performed accurately, and that the teacher will penalize the child by assigning a low homework grade. Ask the teacher to delineate a strategy for evaluating work that has not been completed or performed accurately beyond the identified absolute time limit.

- Discuss with the parents and teacher the demands being imposed on the family as a result of their participation in Homework Success. Families who have trouble with the completion of homework may have particular problems on the evenings they are scheduled to attend Homework Success sessions. Encourage the parents and teacher to identify a strategy to resolve this potential problem.

Goal 5: Enlist the Teacher's Support in Evaluating Program Outcomes

The teacher has a very important role in evaluating the outcomes of Homework Success. The teacher has data pertaining to homework performance that are very useful for progress monitoring and outcome evaluation. Also, the teacher has a wealth of data that is helpful in evaluating the impact of the program on academic functioning.

- Explain to the teacher that Homework Success is a data-based intervention program and that the clinician will be monitoring carefully the child's functioning with homework and schoolwork, as well as the family's functioning, to determine program effects.
- Explain to the teacher the vital role he or she serves in evaluating the effects of Homework Success on homework and academic functioning.
- Ask the teacher to assist in the collection of the following data:

  1. Samples of homework. Ask the teacher to collect and save the child's homework during the course of the program. Ask him or her to begin saving these data immediately. Negotiate a method of reviewing these data on a regular basis to record rates of work completion and accuracy. Emphasize that all homework will be returned to the teacher.
  2. Samples of classwork. Ask the teacher to collect and save the child's classwork beginning immediately. Negotiate a method of reviewing these data on a regular basis.
  3. Teacher records of homework and classwork. Ask the teacher what records are kept regarding homework and classwork performance. Ask him or her if

you can obtain a copy of the child's homework and classwork records on a regular basis.

4. Before leaving, ask the teacher to complete the APQ or the Academic Performance Rating Scale (APRS).

• Close the meeting by identifying specific ways in which the teacher and parents were successful in working collaboratively during the meeting to address the child's homework problems. Encourage the teacher and parents to contact each other with any concerns. Tell them that you will be contacting the teacher regularly to collect data and to review progress. Remind the parents of the time and place of the first parent-training session.

• Thank the teacher and parents for their commitment to collaboration in the child's interests. Make it clear that you are available by telephone to receive feedback and answer questions.

## CHAPTER 7

Group Session 1:
Introducing Homework Success

GOALS:

1. Establish Relationships.
2. Collect baseline data.
3. Introduce program goals and guidelines for group sessions.
4. Educate parents about ADHD and its relation to homework problems.
5. Educate parents about the importance of limiting time spent on homework.
6. Explain the importance of parents completing homework assignments.

This session is primarily designed to set the stage for the sessions that follow by establishing an atmosphere of trust and mutual respect. During this session, parents are informed about the goals and structure of the program. Parents are provided with information about ADHD and the homework problems that are typically associated with this disorder. Parents are instructed about the importance of limiting time spent on homework and using a homework book to record assignments. Clinicians should prepare for this session by having the following materials available:

- The integrity checklist for Session 1 (Appendix C). The integrity checklists outline the steps to follow during each session. These checklists can serve as prompts to clinicians to address the content and process issues pertaining to each session. Clinicians should check each item on the checklist after it has been completed.
- The following handouts (Appendix D):
    Handout 1: Welcome to the Homework Success Program!
    Handout 2: Weekly Family Assignments Sheet
    Handout 3: ADHD: Basic Facts
    Handout 4: Some Ways ADHD Is Related to Homework Problems

Handout 5: Homework Assignment Sheet (with sample)

- The following outcome measures (Appendix B):
  Parent-reported daily logs of work completion, accuracy, and duration
  Conflict Behavior Questionnaire—Parent and Child Forms

GOAL 1: ESTABLISH RELATIONSHIPS

The initial goal is to establish an atmosphere in which parents feel relaxed and are willing to share their ideas and experiences. It is important to begin this session by developing rapport among the clinician and participants. A way to facilitate rapport building is to focus on what the parents have in common—that is, they all have children with attention and learning problems, and they are all coping with a similar set of problems with their children's homework.

- Hand out name tags for each member to wear.
- Introduce yourself to the group. Briefly describe your interest in working with children who have attention and learning problems and your particular interest in helping families cope with homework difficulties.
- Ask participants to introduce themselves and to share their reasons for becoming involved in this program.
- Request that parents talk about one or two problems they have experienced in helping their child with homework.
- As parents state their homework concerns, write them on a chalkboard or dry-erase board for the group to see. Inform parents that they will be addressing the specific problems listed on the board as the program unfolds.
- If a concurrent child-training group is being conducted, encourage the children to introduce themselves and to contribute to the brainstorming discussion. After this part of the session, which should last about 10–15 minutes, the children can be excused to attend their group.

GOAL 2: COMPLETE BASELINE MEASURES

Obtaining baseline data is very important in monitoring progress and evaluating outcomes. Data collected before intervention will serve as a benchmark against which to compare information gathered during intervention and at follow-up. Some baseline data were collected during the initial parent conference. This is a good time to collect additional information.

- Before handing out baseline measures, explain to parents the importance of data collection in assessing progress in homework performance, academic functioning, and family relationships.
- Collect parent-reported daily logs of work completion, accuracy, and duration.

- Distribute the Conflict Behavior Questionnaire–Parent and Child Forms. Ask the parents to complete the parent version. If there is a child group, children can complete the child version measure during Session 1. If not, parents can ask their child to complete this measure and bring it to the next session. Given the nature of the questions on this checklist, the child's responses are more likely to be accurate if they are completed privately by the child. These forms should be returned to group leaders by the next session.

GOAL 3: INTRODUCE PROGRAM GOALS AND GUIDELINES FOR GROUP SESSIONS

Parents need to know about the goals of the program and the format of group sessions. Although this information was introduced during the individualized parent conferences, it should be reviewed in the group. This information will help them to develop realistic expectations for program outcomes, to understand the commitment that is needed from them, and to plan their schedules for the coming weeks. Given that many parents enter programs such as this feeling discouraged, it is important that clinicians introduce the program in a way that instills hope that change is possible if parents make a commitment and follow through with assignments that are given.

During this part of the session, clinicians will begin to distribute handouts to the parents. We encourage clinicians to provide parents with a folder to organize handouts and to model a strategy of organization that may be useful for their children.

- Distribute *Handout 1: Welcome to the Homework Success Program!* (Appendix D).
- Engage parents in a discussion of program goals. Essentially, the goals of Homework Success are to improve homework performance and efficiency, to improve academic functioning, and to build parent–child relationships, thereby reducing parents' stress. Of course, there are many related goals. Parents should be encouraged to generate their own lists. Clinicians can highlight those goals that are most likely to be achieved by making an active commitment to Homework Success.
- Describe the Conjoint Behavioral Consultation model. Key points to present are:

  1. Successful homework intervention requires a collaboration between home and school.
  2. Successful home–school collaboration entails active parental involvement in educational issues and mutual respect between parents and teachers.
  3. The child needs to be an active participant in planning homework interventions.
  4. In solving homework difficulties, the parents, child, and teachers need to assess situations that set children up to fail (antecedents) and consequences for homework behavior that may be maintaining problems.
  5. Interventions should address the antecedents and consequences of homework problems, both in home and school settings.

- Describe the format for the program and for each session.

  1. Weekly meetings are scheduled for 6 weeks, with a follow-up session about 4 weeks after the sixth session.
  2. Each session lasts 90 minutes.
  3. Children have an important role in the intervention process. Describe the way in which children will be included. The structure of a child group that is conducted concurrently with the parent group is described in Chapter 14.
  4. During each session, parents will be given a 10-minute break with refreshments.
  5. A clinician will consult with the child's teacher after the fourth session.

- Present the ground rules for the group.

  1. Prompt and consistent attendance is very important.
  2. The success of the group depends on active participation on the part of each parent.
  3. Participation can be facilitated through active listening by each group member.
  4. Successful home–school collaboration requires that parents communicate frequently and respectfully with teachers.

- Highlight the importance of the parents completing weekly homework assignments. Explain that homework given to the parents will help them to learn and master strategies for helping their child. Further, parental completion of homework assignments models responsible homework behavior for the child.
- Distribute a copy of *Handout 2: Weekly Family Assignment Sheet* (Appendix D) and explain that the parents should complete this at the end of each session when parental homework assignments are given.
- Emphasize that parental homework assignments should be completed by the following session. The assignments will be reviewed and discussed at the beginning of the following session.
- Emphasize the importance of confidentiality and informed consent.

  1. Information shared by parents in the group should not be discussed with persons outside of the group.
  2. Responses to questionnaires completed by parents are held in confidence by clinicians.
  3. Clinicians need to get informed, written consent from parents to obtain and share information about their child with school personnel.

- Acknowledge parental frustration and work to engender hope in families. It is important for clinicians to listen to and empathize with parents regarding the frustrations they experience in raising a child with ADHD or related problems. At the same time, it is critical to emphasize from the outset that Homework Success can make a difference in their family. We encourage clinicians to confidently explain to parents that a strong commitment to the program can result in very positive outcomes. Also, we urge clinicians to express a strong commitment to working with families to resolve unique issues that they face in coping with homework problems.

GOAL 4: EDUCATE PARENTS ABOUT ADHD AND ITS RELATION TO HOMEWORK PROBLEMS

Parents can benefit from education about the problems their child is experiencing and how these problems can have an impact on homework performance, academic functioning, and family relationships. When parents enter treatment for attention and learning problems, they often blame themselves for the difficulties their child is having. Parents need to understand the vulnerabilities of children with ADHD and how deficits in attention and impulse control can lead to homework problems and elicit negative responses from parents. Clinicians should communicate that problems related to ADHD often trigger homework difficulties. At the same time, clinicians should point out that the way that parents respond to their children can serve either to maintain or to resolve problems. Further, educating parents about ADHD and related problems serves to prepare parents for intervention so that they are more ready to invest in the change process.

• Distribute *Handout 3: ADHD: Basic Facts* (Appendix D) and educate parents about ADHD and interventions that are effective in treating this disorder, including the following points:

1. Core dimensions and subtypes.
2. Frequently associated problems (e.g., learning disabilities, defiant behavior, conduct problems, anxiety, and depression).
3. Possible causes.
4. Issues in diagnostic assessment.
5. Effective interventions, including educational, behavioral, and pharmacological.
6. Myths about ADHD.

• As you present information about ADHD, encourage parents to make comments and ask questions.
• Distribute *Handout 4: Some Ways ADHD Is Related to Homework Problems* (Appendix D).
• Refer to the problems written on the board and help parents to understand how ADHD can dispose children to have significant homework difficulties. Explain that children with ADHD often display the following problems with homework:

1. Failure to listen in class and to write down assignments accurately.
2. Tendency to forget to bring home their assignment book and the books needed to complete homework.
3. Unwillingness to begin homework at the appointed time.

4. Failure to sustain attention and persist with work.
5. Frequent distractibility.
6. Lack of productivity.
7. Careless, inaccurate work.
8. Inefficient use of time, often resulting in homework taking much longer than it should.
9. Failure to return assignments to the teacher.

- Elicit parents' comments as you describe how ADHD disposes children to display these problems.

GOAL 5: EDUCATE PARENTS ABOUT THE IMPORTANCE OF LIMITING TIME SPENT ON HOMEWORK

Children with ADHD and their families typically spend an excessive amount of time completing homework, resulting in frustration and conflictual parent–child interactions. Putting limits on the amount of time spent doing homework can help to make homework more manageable and productive, break the cycle of family conflict, and bring about more frequent experiences of success. As such, it is recommended that daily time spent on homework be limited to a specific amount of time. At the parent–teacher conference held before this meeting, teachers should have specified the absolute time limit for children to spend on their homework each day. Many parents find it difficult to place limits on homework time, because they are concerned that teachers will not understand, that teachers will evaluate homework performance more negatively, and that grades in school could be affected. Clinicians must be prepared to address these parental concerns when recommending a reduction in homework time.

- Explain to parents the problems that can arise when children spend long amounts of time doing homework. Describe how extended homework sessions can lead to wasted time, frustration to the child, frustration to the parent, parental reinforcement of unproductive behavior, parent–child conflict, and failure to address other family issues, including time spent with a spouse or siblings.
- Help parents to understand that there is a point beyond which there is no return for the investment of additional time spent doing homework. In fact, when homework exceeds a certain amount of time, it can have very negative side effects.
- Describe the benefits of limiting homework time, which include:

1. Teaching children to work more efficiently.
2. Enabling children to become more responsible by experiencing the consequences of their inefficiency.
3. Reducing the occasions for parental reprimands and conflictual parent–child exchanges.
4. Reducing the period of time that parents need to focus energy on helping their child with homework, thereby freeing parents to attend to other family matters.

- Inform parents that general guidelines have been established to determine the point of diminishing returns with homework. Present the following guidelines as upper limits for homework time:

Grade 1:	30 minutes
Grades 2–3:	60 minutes
Grades 4–6:	90 minutes

- Acknowledge that these guidelines err on the side of giving the child more time than most teachers will require.
- Encourage parents to share the progress they made with their child's teachers in delineating the maximum amount of time to be spent doing homework each day.
- Instruct the parents not to provide any additional assistance to children after the time limit for homework has expired. Parents should inform the child that homework time is over and that they are not going to provide any additional help. After the time limit has expired, the parent can permit the child to work independently on homework if the child wants to do so. However, it is very important that the parent not get drawn back into issues pertaining to homework.
- Encourage parents to express their misgivings about this strategy. A common concern is that children will complete only a portion of their work. Parents worry what teachers will think and how their child's homework will be evaluated. For this reason, it is critical for parents to collaborate with the teacher so that the teacher endorses this strategy and does not penalize the child for incomplete work during the initial stages of intervention.

GOAL 6: IMPLEMENT A TOOL FOR RECORDING HOMEWORK ASSIGNMENTS

A very common problem, particularly for children with ADHD, is the failure to accurately record homework assignments. When a child does not write down assignments correctly, it makes it very difficult for parents to provide assistance and to hold the child accountable for completing work. Developing a tool to help children record assignments is a critical step for improving homework performance.

- Discuss with parents the importance of a homework assignment book. Explain that the assignment book serves not only as a reminder to students but also as a tool parents can use to verify that homework has been completed.
- Encourage parents to talk about the progress they made in discussing with their child's teacher a method for ensuring that homework assignments are recorded accurately.
- Distribute *Handout 5: Homework Assignment Sheet* (Appendix D), including the sample completed assignment sheet. Explain to parents how this sheet should be used. Most students already use a homework assignment book. If this is the case, the child can continue to use his or her current assignment book. It is critical in this intervention to have an entry for each subject. If there is no homework for a particular subject, the

child should write "NA" for "no assignment." For the child who often fails to record assignments correctly, it is also essential that the teacher check the homework book and initial it if the assignments are written down accurately. For students who have only one teacher, it is sufficient for the teacher to check the homework book at the end of the school day. For children who have several teachers, it is critical that they have the homework book checked at the end of each class period.

HOMEWORK ASSIGNMENTS FOR PARENTS

The primary homework assignments are to make sure that the homework assignment book is being used consistently and accurately on a daily basis and to enforce the absolute time limits established during the parent–teacher meeting. Also, parents need to continue recording data regarding work completion, accuracy, and duration.

- Ask the parents to record their homework assignments on *Handout 2: Weekly Family Assignment Sheet.*
- Request that the parents finalize a method for their child to record homework assignments. Tell parents that they may need to confer with the teacher to ensure that assignments are written accurately and clearly. In most cases, it will be necessary for the teacher to check and initial the homework assignment book. Instruct the parents to bring the homework book to each session.
- Ask the parents to rigidly enforce the absolute time limit for homework established at the parent–teacher meeting. Remind the parents not to assist the child with homework after the absolute time limit has expired.
- Request that the parents fill in the logs of homework completion, accuracy, and duration every day and submit these logs at the following session.

CHAPTER 8

Group Session 2: Establishing a Homework Ritual and Giving Instructions

]GOALS

1. Review homework
2. Assist parents in analyzing the antecedents and consequences of behavior.
3. Assist parents in establishing a homework ritual.
4. Educate parents about giving instructions to their child.

This session is designed to provide a framework for the behavioral strategies that are introduced throughout the program. Participants are taught to identify and specify a target behavior and to examine environmental events that have occurred before and after the behavior that may be serving to trigger or maintain problems. Parents are instructed to use a strategy, the Homework A-B-Cs, to analyze antecedent events and consequences that may be contributing to homework problems. This session focuses primarily on examining and changing the antecedents of problematic behavior. Parents are directed to reflect on the ground rules for homework that are currently being applied, including issues pertaining to the time and place for homework. Guidelines for redesigning the homework ritual are provided. Further, parents are requested to examine how they give instructions and commands to their child. Specific guidelines for giving effective instructions to children are outlined. Clinicians should prepare for this session by having the following materials available:

- The integrity checklist for Session 2 (Appendix C). Clinicians should check each item on the checklist after it has been completed.
- The following handouts (Appendix D):
  Handout 6: *Homework A-B-C Worksheet*

Handout 7: *Establishing the Homework Ritual*
Handout 8: *Homework Ritual Worksheet*
Handout 9: *Effective Instructions*

- The following outcome measures (Appendix B):
Homework Performance Questionnaire
Homework Success Evaluation Inventory

GOAL 1: REVIEW HOMEWORK

Reviewing homework provides immediate feedback to parents about their work and reinforces the importance of their completing assignments and doing so on time. Reviewing homework also enables the clinician to monitor progress, to identify assignments that were difficult for parents, and to provide guidance to parents. The review of homework during this session consists primarily of monitoring the child's progress in completing the homework assignment book and the parents' success in implementing an absolute time limit for homework.

- Ask parents to complete the Homework Performance Questionnaire and Homework Success Evaluation Inventory before reviewing homework.
- Request that parents submit their daily logs of homework performance.
- Ask parents to share their child's homework assignment book. Check to see that the assignment book is being used daily and that teachers are checking and initialing entries into this book.
- Ask parents to report on their initial experiences using a homework assignment book. Once again, focus primarily on parents' successes in using this intervention. Identify problems that have arisen and encourage the group to help each other in problem solving.
- Ask parents to report on the conversation they had with their child about homework concerns. Ask them to list the concerns that their child identified. Write these problems on newsprint or the chalkboard for reference later in the session.
- Ask parents to report on their experiences in implementing absolute time limits for homework. Many parents encounter significant problems applying this intervention because they are so fearful that their child will not complete work and will be evaluated negatively by the teacher. Stress the importance of adhering to time limits and not helping their child with homework issues after the time limit has expired. It is often useful to suggest that parents use a countdown timer to enforce time limits.

GOAL 2: ASSIST PARENTS IN ANALYZING THE ANTECEDENTS AND CONSEQUENCES OF BEHAVIOR

Parents typically enter a program like this believing that they are to blame for many of the homework problems their child is demonstrating. It is important to reassure parents that problems with homework have many causes and that one important factor is that their child has strong, intrinsic tendencies to have difficulty with homework. At the same time, parents need to understand that the way in which the homework environment is organized and the way they respond to their child's behavior are strong contributing factors to these problems. A strategy is introduced to the parents to help them specify problem behaviors and identify antecedent events and consequences that may be triggering and maintaining the targeted behaviors.

- Elicit from parents some of the factors that cause children's behavior problems. Examples might include a biologically based disposition to be inattentive and impulsive, a child's lack of sleep, worry about a problem with peer relationships, and ineffective parenting practices.
- Emphasize that behavior problems have multiple causes but that environmental events that precede and follow behavior are particularly important because they have the greatest chance of being altered. Provide parents with examples of antecedent events that can trigger problem behaviors (e.g., allowing a child do homework in front of the television may make it difficult for the child to concentrate and be productive). Provide the parents with examples of consequences that can maintain irresponsibility on the part of the child (e.g., allowing the child to watch television when homework has not been completed will maintain unproductive behavior).
- Distribute *Handout 6: Homework A-B-C Worksheet*. Explain to parents that "A" refers to antecedents, "B" refers to behavior, and "C" refers to Consequences.
- Ask a parent to volunteer to do a functional assessment of a homework difficulty that arose during the previous week. It may be useful to refer to the list of problems written on the board. Ask the parents to describe environmental events that preceded the occurrence of the targeted behavior. Encourage participants to identify which of these environmental events may have triggered the problem. Also ask the parents to describe events that took place during and after the child's problematic behavior, with a particular focus on the parents' response to the child's behavior. Encourage participants to identify consequences that may be maintaining the problem.
- Ask each parent to perform a functional assessment of a homework difficulty using the A-B-C Worksheet. Review one or two of these after the parents have completed this exercise.

GOAL 3: ASSIST PARENTS IN ESTABLISHING A HOMEWORK RITUAL

For the remainder of this session, parents will focus on changing the antecedents of homework behavior as a way of triggering more attentive and productive responding. Parents are encouraged to examine the context within which their child completes homework—more specifically, the where, when, and what of homework, which we refer to as the homework ritual. Because children with ADHD typically have significant problems with organization and because they are often highly task avoidant, it is particularly important to focus on establishing a sound homework ritual for these individuals.

- Distribute *Handout 7: Establishing the Homework Ritual.*
- Describe the importance of doing homework in a location that is conducive to attentive and productive work. Ask the parents to describe the location in which their child does homework and encourage them to examine the extent to which this place promotes productive behavior.
- Emphasize to parents the importance of designating a location for homework that minimizes distractions and is situated where a parent can readily provide ongoing supervision.
- Describe the importance of doing homework at the right time. Ask parents what time their child does his or her homework and encourage the parents to analyze the extent to which their child is working at a time that promotes attentive behavior.
- Emphasize to parents the importance of selecting a time for homework that maximizes the child's ability to pay attention and the parents' ability to monitor homework performance. Parents often ask whether it is better to do homework right after school or to wait for a while. The answer to this question depends on the child's ability to pay attention and the parents' ability to supervise homework.
- Stress that it is important, if possible, to select a consistent time to begin homework. Having a consistent time will help to establish a reasonable expectation for the start of homework and prevent the child from perceiving the parent as being arbitrary in deciding when homework should begin.
- Indicate that homework should be divided into units of work, with each unit generally corresponding to an assignment in a particular subject. The child can be given a break after each unit of work, but it is important that the break be very short (1–2 minutes) so that it is easy for the child to become reengaged with work.
- Emphasize the importance of the child being organized and prepared to do work. To complete work and minimize wasted time, children need to have their homework assignment book, books, and worksheets, and homework supplies in front of them. Encourage the parents to spend time with their child putting together a homework kit with the supplies needed to do most homework assignments.
- Distribute *Handout 8: Homework Ritual Worksheet.* Make sure the parents understand this worksheet and tell the parents that they will be asked to work with their child in completing this worksheet as a homework assignment.

GOAL 4: EDUCATE PARENTS ABOUT GIVING INSTRUCTIONS TO THEIR CHILD

Another set of environmental events that can promote attentive and productive behavior is the way in which parents issue instructions to their child. If instructions are issued properly, children are quite likely to follow through and be compliant. In contrast, instructions that are issued improperly, something that often occurs when parents are frustrated, typically are ineffective. Parents can benefit greatly from guidelines about how to issue instructions in a manner that is clear, concise, and reasonable.

- Distribute *Handout 9: Effective Instructions.*
- Review the characteristics of effective instructions:

1. Minimize distractions. For example, television is a frequent distracter when parents are issuing instructions. If the child is looking at the television when you need to give an instruction, stand between the child and the television when making a request.

2. Try to maintain eye contact with the child when giving an instruction.

3. Make brief requests that focus on one specific behavior at a time. For example, instead of saying, "Turn off the television, get your homework kit, get your book bag, and go to the bathroom before getting started with homework," it would be better to issue one instruction at a time and to praise the child for each act of compliance.

4. Issue the instruction as a statement. In other words, do not state requests in terms of a question or a favor to you. Examples of all three are:
   Question: Could you start your homework now?
   Favor: Would you do me a favor and get started with your homework now?
   Statement: You need to start your homework now.

5. Offer instructions that are reasonable and achievable. Avoid giving instructions that set children up to fail. For example, instead of saying, "Finish your homework, then study spelling, and then do your book report," it would be better to issue a more specific and realistic statement: "Let's work to complete the problems on this page in the next 10 minutes."

6. Verify that the child has heard and understood the instruction. The easiest way to do this is to check to see if the child is implementing the task he or she was instructed to perform. Another way to do this is to ask the child to repeat the instruction. However, if he or she becomes frustrated or defiant when asked to repeat the instruction, then this technique should not be used.

7. Make sure you mean what you say and are ready to follow up if the child does not follow through with the instruction. After you offer a command, watch what the child does and offer consequences based on his or her actions.

8. Make clear to the child how many times you are willing to repeat a command before you will implement a consequence. Our recommendation is to make a request, wait 15 seconds, issue a warning, and then provide a consequence within 5 additional seconds if the child does not follow through.

9. Provide praise when your child begins to follow through with your directions. Don't wait for your child to complete a task before issuing praise. The child is more likely to follow through if you provide praise for his or her initial attempts to comply.

• Invite parents to discuss these points as you are presenting them. Encourage parents to identify obstacles to issuing clear, concise, reasonable instructions to their child.

HOMEWORK ASSIGNMENTS FOR PARENTS

The following homework assignments are given to parents as an opportunity for them to collaborate with their child and to practice the strategies covered during this session.

Remind parents to write down their assignments on the Weekly Family Assignment Sheet.

- Request that the parents identify at least three problematic homework behaviors and complete the Homework A-B-C exercise for each of these behaviors.
- Ask the parents to collaborate with their child to establish the homework ritual. Request that they complete the Homework Ritual Worksheet.
- Request that the parents and child post the homework ritual in a prominent place close to where the child completes homework.
- Request that the parents follow the guidelines outlined in this session when issuing instructions to their child.
- Ask the parents to praise their child when he or she begins to follow through on instructions.
- Remind parents to bring in their child's homework assignment book the following week.
- Remind the parents to keep filling out the daily logs of homework completion, accuracy, and duration.

OBTAINING OUTCOME DATA FROM THE TEACHER

After this session, contact the teacher and make arrangements to collect outcome data. Specifically, ask the teacher to (1) complete the Academic Performance Rating Scale (APRS), (2) submit samples of the child's homework and classwork, and (3) submit copies of records of homework, classwork, and test performance. If the teacher is busy and will have trouble compiling these materials, offer assistance with photocopying, if appropriate. Ask the teacher to comment on the child's progress and to identify problems that still need to be addressed. Thank the teacher for investing in the program and supporting the parents.

CHAPTER 9

Group Session 3:
Providing Positive Reinforcement

GOALS

1. Review homework.
2. Elicit examples of positive reinforcement.
3. Explain rationale for positive reinforcement.
4. Present types of positive reinforcers.
5. Assist parents in developing an individualized positive reinforcement system.
6. Underscore the central components of positive reinforcement.

The primary goal of this session is to train parents in the principles and techniques of positive reinforcement. This session emphasizes the use of consequences within the A-B-C model to increase desired behaviors. The technique of positive reinforcement is discussed relatively early in the program so as to emphasize the importance of using a positive approach to address children's behavior problems and to allow time throughout the group for parents to practice these critical skills.

During this session, the clinician elicits and acknowledges the difficulties parents have experienced in attempting to identify and reinforce positive behaviors in a child with ADHD. Specific types of reinforcers are described, including parental attention, praise, privileges, and concrete rewards. The clinician provides guidance to the parents in planning a token reinforcement program with their child. In addition, the core components of reinforcement are described through the acronym CISS-4, which refers to Consistency, Immediacy, Specificity, Saliency, and a 4:1 ratio of positive-to-negative responses to children's behaviors. The clinician discusses the rationale and means of implementing each of these elements of an effective system of positive reinforcement. Clinicians should prepare for this session by preparing the following materials:

- The integrity checklist for Session 3 (Appendix C).
- The following handouts (Appendix D):
  Handout 10: Using Positive Reinforcement
  Handout 11: Homework Rewards Worksheet (with sample)
  Handout 12: Token and Point System Guidelines

GOAL 1: REVIEW HOMEWORK

To emphasize the importance of completing Homework Success assignments, homework given at the conclusion of the previous session should be reviewed. The review of homework also serves to provide parents with feedback regarding assignments that were challenging to them. Through the discussion of the homework ritual, the A-B-C exercise, and guidelines for delivering instructions, clinicians have the opportunity to highlight once again the importance of focusing on antecedents in changing children's behavior.

- Collect parent-reported logs of work completion, accuracy, and duration.
- Review each child's homework assignment book.
- Ask parents to describe the discussions they had with their child pertaining to the homework ritual. Focus on and emphasize strategies used by the parents that elicited involvement and cooperation from their child. Assist the parents in finalizing their plan for establishing the time and place for homework.
- Ask parents to discuss their experiences in delivering instructions to their child. Specifically, encourage them to provide examples of both effective and ineffective commands that they issued since the last session. Encourage group members to provide assistance to parents who have had trouble delivering effective instructions.
- Encourage parents to discuss the Homework A-B-C exercise. Specifically, ask parents about antecedents to problem behaviors that they have identified and recorded over the past week. Also, ask them to discuss any changes they made in the antecedents and their child's response to these modifications. Collect the Homework A-B-C Worksheet from the parents after this discussion.
- When parents do not or only partially comply with between-session assignments, specify what the parents did accomplish and provide verbal praise for these behaviors. Such an approach increases the likelihood that they will do homework in the future and models for parents the importance of focusing on and reinforcing desired, responsible behaviors. Also, review the rationale for having parents complete assignments: First, strategies presented are unlikely to be effective if parents and children do not implement and practice them to the point at which the interventions become part of their routine; and, second, group leaders can help parents to refine their strategies if they come to the group prepared to discuss their experiences in implementing the techniques at home. Further, it is often useful to engage parents in a brief dialogue regarding barriers to the implementation of assignments. Once barriers have been identified, group members can be invited to share strategies for overcoming these obstacles.

GOAL 2: ELICIT EXAMPLES OF POSITIVE REINFORCEMENT

Parents often enter the group feeling quite frustrated and focusing primarily on their child's irresponsible and unproductive behaviors. Parents generally require much encouragement to focus on their child's positive behaviors. At the same time, it is important to acknowledge the good work that they are already doing in reinforcing their children's responsible behaviors.

• Ask parents to report two or three times in the previous week when they acknowledged their child's responsible and cooperative behavior. Identify the specific ways in which parents reinforced their child's adaptive behavior. Praise the parents for their efforts to selectively attend to their child's responsible behaviors.
• Refer to these examples as you provide the rationale and description of the use of positive reinforcement.

GOAL 3: EXPLAIN RATIONALE FOR POSITIVE REINFORCEMENT

It is critical that parents understand the importance of using positive reinforcement as a method to change their child's behavior. Many parents enter groups such as these expecting to learn about methods of punishment, so it is important to explain to parents why we focus on reinforcing responsible behavior before addressing punitive strategies. Also, it is important to acknowledge that many parents have trouble using positive reinforcement strategies and to understand the problems parents have had implementing these techniques in the past.

• Distribute *Handout 10: Using Positive Reinforcement*.
• Discuss the principles of and rationale for positive reinforcement. Specifically, address the following main points:

1. Positive reinforcement is a consequence of behavior that increases the likelihood that the behavior will reoccur. A consequence that does not increase the probability of a specified behavior occurring is not a positive reinforcer, even if the consequence seems to be something that a person wants. Elicit examples from the parents (e.g., dessert after dinner may seem to be a positive reinforcer for a child, but if the child does not elicit responsible eating behavior in an effort to get dessert, then this consequence may not be reinforcing for the child). Also, a consequence that may appear to be adverse to a child may actually be positively reinforcing. A common example is how parental reprimands often result in an increase in disruptive behavior.
2. Delivering positive reinforcement in response to a desired behavior and not providing positive reinforcement for an undesired behavior is a very effective behavior change strategy. Provide examples to the parents (e.g., supervisors at work can have a significant impact on their employees by praising certain behaviors and not praising other actions).

- Emphasize the importance of focusing on positive reinforcement strategies before focusing on other methods, such as punishment. Positive reinforcement strategies are much more effective than punishment techniques in promoting skill development. Also, positive reinforcement methods help to develop self-esteem in children. In contrast, punishment can be associated with negative side effects if it is not embedded in a primarily positive system of contingency management.

- Discuss with parents the reasons why it can be so difficult to implement positive reinforcement strategies.

1. Children with ADHD often display high rates of uncooperative and unproductive behaviors. Parents may develop a habit of focusing primarily on the maladaptive behaviors because they are so frequent and salient. Many parents have a difficult time focusing on responsible behaviors because they seem to occur so infrequently. In these cases, it is critical for parents to vigilantly look for and acknowledge their child's responsible behaviors, even when examples of such behavior do not seem to occur very often.

2. Parents often hold beliefs that do not promote the frequent and consistent use of positive reinforcement. For instance, many parents expect their child to be responsible and do not believe children should be rewarded for what is expected of them. Although this attitude is understandable, it often leads to parental behavior that is overly critical and punitive. Help the parents understand that any approach to parenting that results in disproportionately high (over 20% of the feedback given to children) rates of punitive consequences may not be effective and may result in negative side effects, such as increased defiance and a deterioration of the parent–child relationship. Encourage parents to acknowledge their child's starting point and to work toward gradually changing behavior.

3. Parents often believe that a child will begin to act out if they identify and reinforce adaptive behaviors. Acknowledge that a child may become inattentive and disruptive after a parent provides attention and praise but that parental attention to productive behavior is not the reason for the problem. Encourage parents to evaluate a sample situation using the A-B-C system. For example, the child is working attentively at homework. The parent notices the child's productive behavior and provides praise. The child then looks away from her work and speaks to the parent. The parent tells the child to get back to work, and the child engages with the parent in an argument. Through an analysis of this situation, help the parents to see that it is not parental praise of productive behavior that maintains the problem but the parent's response to the child's attention-seeking, inattentive behavior after praise is provided that reinforces and maintains the child's unproductive, argumentative behavior.

GOAL 4: PRESENT TYPES OF POSITIVE REINFORCERS

A positive reinforcement system involves attending to desirable behaviors and applying a reinforcer that is appropriate for a child's level of development and that is effective in changing the child's behavior. Some parents have concerns about using concrete objects such as toys and food to reinforce their child. This section will help to address some parental concerns about the types of consequences used as reinforcers.

- Provide an overview of the various types of positive reinforcers, including the following:

    1. *Sense of personal pride,* referring to the intrinsic reward of performing a behavior that results in a sense of accomplishment.
    2. *Attention,* referring to the involvement of adults or peers with a child in response to a specific behavior. Attention can be provided in verbal and nonverbal ways and can involve praise, criticism, or neutral behavior toward a child. Ask parents to provide examples of how verbal and nonverbal demonstrations of attention can be used as positive reinforcers (e.g., conversing with a child during homework may positively reinforce the behavior occurring at the time of the discussion).
    3. *Praise,* referring to complimentary feedback offered to a child in response to a desired behavior. Praise can be provided in both verbal and nonverbal ways. Encourage parents to describe their favorite ways of providing verbal and nonverbal praise to their child.
    4. *Privileges,* referring to access to special activities contingent on performing a desired behavior. Once again, encourage parents to provide examples of privileges that can be used as reinforcers in their home (e.g., later bedtime, television show, access to the internet).
    5. *Concrete rewards,* referring to materials provided to a child in response to specified, targeted behaviors. Examples of concrete rewards include toys, stickers, food, and money. Explain to parents that concrete rewards are the least preferred types of reinforcers because of the expense and the possibility of conditioning children to expect material objects for desirable behavior. Nonetheless, concrete rewards can have powerful effects on children and can be very useful when behavior is difficult to change.

- Explain to parents that the various reinforcer types exist on a hierarchy, with intrinsic motivation being the most preferred and concrete rewards being the least preferred. In selecting a reinforcer, it is recommended that parents use consequences at the highest level of the hierarchy that is effective in changing behavior. Stress to parents that the highest effective level of reinforcement will be different for each child and family. Also, indicate that each child may show great variability in responding to different types of reinforcers. To illustrate the latter point, group leaders may wish to use examples or to elicit some examples from parents. For instance, a child may take genuine pride (i.e., upper end of the hierarchy) in scoring highly on a video game, but the same child may require concrete rewards (i.e., lower end of the hierarchy) to persist in completing a homework assignment.

GOAL 5: ASSIST PARENTS IN DEVELOPING AN INDIVIDUALIZED POSITIVE REINFORCEMENT SYSTEM

Token reinforcement is a method of providing salient positive reinforcement to children in a way that is easy and efficient for parents to use. An added advantage is that tokens and points can be provided immediately after desirable behaviors occur. Most parents have some understanding of token reinforcement systems already. During this section, clinicians can help parents to refine their knowledge of this technique and to consider ways of applying the strategy at home with their child.

• Introduce the concept of a token reinforcement system, that is, an approach similar to a monetary system whereby children earn tokens or points for desired behavior that can be exchanged at some time in the future for a privilege or concrete reward. Discuss with parents the notion that for many children with ADHD, personal pride (i.e., self-reinforcement) and praise from parents are not sufficiently powerful reinforcers to result in significant improvements in homework performance.

• Describe the rationale for using a token/point reinforcement system:

1. Token systems enable parents to strengthen the reinforcement they provide, which can make behavior modification systems more effective.

2. Token systems provide parents with a tool to respond immediately to a child's desirable behavior. These systems are easy to use. Parents can dispense tokens and points very readily at the time their child exhibits the desired behavior.

3. Token systems provide a means of reinforcing children that is affordable to most families. Instead of giving children relatively expensive items each time they exhibit the targeted behaviors, parents can provide children with tokens or points that can be stored and cashed in at some later time. Relatedly, it is feasible to dispense tokens on a frequent basis, enabling a parent to reinforce targeted behavior as often as needed.

4. These systems may help children learn to work for long-term reinforcers. This is particularly relevant for children with ADHD, who tend to have difficulty delaying gratification. Tokens provide a measure of immediate reinforcement but also orient children to work for longer term goals and reinforcers.

• Distribute *Handout 12: Token and Point System Guidelines*. Review these instructions for implementing a token and point reinforcement system with the parents.

1. Parents need to determine whether they will use poker chips, tokens, or points with their children. Older children, or those with relatively mild ADHD, may respond well to the use of points. Conversely, younger children and those with more severe ADHD symptoms will generally require the use of more concrete objects, such as tokens or chips.

2. If it is determined that tokens or chips will be used, some practical issues must be considered. For instance, parents may wish to consider purchasing an attractive receptacle for earned tokens to increase the child's interest in

the system. Alternately, parents may decide to construct a receptacle with the child when introducing the system. If poker chips are used, points can be assigned to them depending on color. For instance, blue chips may be worth 10 points, red chips 5 points, and white chips 1 point. Chips can be taped to a small card with points written below them.

3. Parents need to sit down with their child and discuss the program. We suggest that the system be introduced to children as a means of rewarding their homework efforts. This way the system is introduced in a positive manner.

4. Describe the use of a reward menu, which is a list of rewards that the child can choose from when a reinforcer is earned. Emphasize that the process of creating a reward menu involves negotiation between the parent and child. To this end, the parent should be discouraged from criticizing or otherwise evaluating reward ideas offered by the child. Acknowledge that some children may suggest items or activities that are relatively expensive or time-consuming. Some parents become concerned when children select relatively expensive rewards. Of course, there are limits to what parents can afford to buy their child, but remind parents that token reinforcement systems are particularly suited to this type of problem. Children can be required to earn a large number of tokens in order to attain these more expensive reinforcers. Also, clinicians should encourage parents to develop a list of reinforcers that includes less expensive items or less time-consuming privileges.

5. Parents should clearly outline for the child the tasks needed to earn the rewards. Include tasks that are relatively difficult (e.g., bringing home the assignment book with the required signatures; starting homework on time), as well as those that are relatively easy for the child (e.g., having pencils sharpened when starting homework).

6. The number of chips or points required for each reinforcer should be specified. Parents should err on the side of being generous to the child in assigning point values for reinforcers, particularly when the system is in its initial stages of usage.

7. Remind parents to focus primarily on positive behaviors. As noted on the rewards worksheet, bonus points should be given for exceptional behaviors and the child's cooperation with the system.

8. Stress to parents that reinforcers should be frequently varied to maintain the child's investment. A number of strategies can be used to help vary the reinforcers provided to a child. For instance, parents can use a grab bag; when the child earns a reinforcer, he or she can reach into a bag of small toys and pick one out. Alternately, the child can roll dice or spin a wheel when a reinforcer is earned. A different reinforcer can be assigned to each number on the dice or wheel. Still another idea is to use a mystery motivator, whereby the parent writes down the reinforcer on an index card and places it an envelope that is taped high on the wall near the homework location. When the reinforcement criterion is reached, the child is able to get the envelope and receive the reinforcer indicated.

9. Assist parents in devising a method to keep track of tokens or points earned

for each of the targeted behaviors. Distribute *Handout 11: Homework Rewards Worksheet*. This worksheet specifies possible targets for intervention and provides spaces for indicating points earned for each behavior each day. The sample *Homework Rewards Worksheet* provides an example of how this technique can be used.

10. Emphasize to parents that, although tokens and points are distributed frequently, reinforcers are to be given only after homework is completed and only if they have been earned. The latter point is particularly important, as some children will attempt to bargain with the parent (e.g., "I promise to do better tomorrow; just please give me the reward tonight."). Group leaders should instruct parents that if a reinforcer is not earned, they should not criticize the child but should express their hope that a reward will be earned during the next homework session.

11. As a related point, remind parents that the system should be devised to ensure that the child earns a reward approximately 80% of the time. Note that if the child succeeds less than 80% of the time, both the child and parent may become discouraged and discontinue the system. Alternately, if reinforcers are too readily earned, the incentive to improve behaviors may be weakened.

12. Parents should be encouraged to have the child actually deposit the tokens or chips in the fabricated bank or to enter points in the point book, as the physical act of doing so may promote the child's investment in this reinforcement system.

13. As with most of the interventions introduced in the Homework Success Program, clinicians should counsel patience. Acknowledge that some children may display oppositional behaviors, particularly when the system is initially being implemented. Some children may even fail to earn reinforcers for several days. However, encourage parents to be patient, persistent, and consistent in their use of the system, as most children ultimately find the experience to be a positive and enjoyable one.

14. Suggest that parents include their child's siblings (if any) in the reinforcement system, but emphasize that parents must be careful to individualize the system so that it is responsive to the developmental level of each child.

• As you explain the components of a token reinforcement system, encourage the parents to ask questions and make comments. It is important for parents to leave this session with a good idea about how to implement a token system.

GOAL 6: UNDERSCORE THE CENTRAL COMPONENTS OF POSITIVE REINFORCEMENT

During this session, a high volume of information has been conveyed to the parents. It is very important that they identify and remember key points about the use of positive reinforcement. We have devised the acronym "CISS-4" to help parents recall the critical elements of positive reinforcement.

- *Consistency.* Emphasize that it is important that children know what responses to expect when they behave in a desirable or undesirable manner. In other words, they need to be able to predict consequences when they display certain behaviors. Therefore, it is important that parents respond in the same way when children display a given set of behaviors. When parents are consistent about what behaviors they want, children know what is expected of them. Acknowledge that consistency is often simpler to discuss than to display. However, group leaders should emphasize that the techniques of this program, such as the token/point system, facilitate consistency.

- *Immediacy.* It is important to reinforce desirable behaviors as immediately as possible after they occur to ensure that the child understands the connection between his or her behavior and the parent's response. Explain that the closer the timing between the child's behavior and its consequence, the greater the chance of the child learning to behave in the desired manner. Acknowledge that certain reinforcers (e.g., privileges) cannot always be administered immediately. However, it should be stressed that the token/point system provides a mechanism for the parent to provide salient positive feedback to the child immediately.

- *Specificity.* Emphasize the importance of being specific about exactly which behaviors are being reinforced. Being specific about the behaviors being reinforced serves the goal of strengthening the connection between responsible behaviors and desirable consequences, thereby resulting in an increased likelihood that the targeted behaviors will be repeated. Provide an example of a nonspecific versus a specific statement. A nonspecific statement is, "I am letting you stay up late because you were good." A specific statement is, "I am letting you stay up until 10:00 P.M. because you finished the chapter in your science book."

- *Saliency.* Note that reinforcers are more likely to be effective in changing behavior if they are highly valuable to the child. As indicated earlier, it is often necessary to vary reinforcers to keep them meaningful to the child.

- *4:1 ratio of positive reinforcement to punishment.* In order for a behavioral system to be effective, it is important that the child experience success at least 80% of the time. Explain that it is easy for parents to revert to the habit of focusing on irresponsible behaviors, because these are so salient and at times annoying. Because it is so easy to ignore productive behaviors, it is important to make a special effort to identify and reinforce responsible behaviors, however minor or seemingly trivial. A ratio of at least 4:1 positive-reinforcement-to-punishment responses not only is effective but also ensures that children experience high rates of success, which will enhance their self-esteem and sense of competence. Note that primarily positive responses from parents can also improve the parent–child relationship.

HOMEWORK ASSIGNMENTS FOR PARENTS

The following homework assignments are given as an opportunity for parents to implement and practice the skills addressed during this session. Remind the parents to write down their assignments on the Weekly Family Assignment Sheet.

- Request that the parents meet with their child to devise a token reinforcement program. Emphasize the importance of developing the following components of the system:

    1. *Reward menu.* The parents and child should create a menu of reinforcers that includes various reinforcer types, with a particular focus on privileges. Parents should encourage their child to suggest reinforcers of varying levels of expense.
    2. *Identifying homework tasks.* The parents and child should develop a list of homework tasks. Encourage the parents to include tasks that vary in level of difficulty.
    3. *Assigning point values.* The parents and child should determine point values for each homework task, with more difficult tasks earning a higher number of points.

- Request that the parents work with their child to create a chart that clearly identifies the reward menu, the homework tasks, and the point values for completing each task. This chart should be posted in a prominent place near the homework location.
- Request that the parents begin implementing the token system. Refer the parents to the guidelines in Handout 12. Emphasize the importance of being patient during the initial stages of implementation.
- Give parents several additional A-B-C Worksheets and request that they continue to complete these logs whenever a problematic homework situation arises. Request that they complete this sheet at least twice in the coming week.
- Remind the parents to continue filling out the daily parent logs of homework completion, accuracy, and duration.
- Encourage parents to call you if any questions or concerns arise in the coming week.

CHAPTER 10

Group Session 4: Managing Time and Setting Goals

GOALS

1. Review homework.
2. Describe the importance of time management and goal setting.
3. Provide instruction in how to manage time and set goals.

If any single session can be said to be at the very core of the Homework Success Program, it is Session 4. This session brings together elements of parent behavioral training and child self-management of homework, both of which have received support in the research literature. More specifically, improvements in academic performance have been demonstrated when children (1) actively participate in goal setting, (2) engage in self-evaluations of performance, (3) receive feedback regarding performance, and (4) are provided with positive reinforcers that are contingent upon meeting goals. All of these components are included in the curriculum for this session.

Learning how to use time-management and goal-setting techniques can be a somewhat complex process for parents. Therefore, clinicians should devote particular attention to ensuring that parents fully understand and receive support in practicing each step of the goal-setting strategies. Although the handout that accompanies this session provides clear, step-by-step directions for time management and goal setting, group leaders need to support parents regarding consistent use of the techniques and to help in troubleshooting problems. Clinicians should have the following materials prepared for this session:

- The integrity checklist for Session 4 (Appendix C).
- The following handout (Appendix D):
  Handout 13: Managing Time and Goal Setting

- The following outcome measures (Appendix B):
  Homework Performance Questionnaire
  Homework Success Evaluation Inventory

GOAL 1: REVIEW HOMEWORK

Parents need immediate feedback on their performance with homework assignments to reinforce the importance of completing assigned tasks and to provide guidance with components that are challenging for them. Homework assigned at the last session, in particular the task of developing a token reinforcement system with their child, is a complex and challenging activity. Clinicians may need to spend more time reviewing homework during this session than they have for the previous sessions.

- Collect parent-reported logs of homework completion, accuracy, and duration.
- Request that parents complete the Homework Performance Questionnaire and Homework Success Evaluation Inventory.
- Discuss parents' experiences in planning a token reinforcement system with their child. Identify elements of the planning process that were successful, and encourage parents to offer praise to one another. Ask parents to report on their progress in developing a reward menu, in identifying tasks to be completed during homework, and in assigning point or token values to each task. Provide guidance to parents in addressing each of these critical elements of a token system.
- Discuss parents' experiences with the implementation of the token system. In doing so, we suggest that clinicians ask each set of parents to complete the A-B-C Worksheet. Ask parents to identify the behavior targeted for change. Request that they identify an occasion on which their child demonstrated the target behavior and they used the token system. Have them identify the antecedents, behavior, consequence (provision of tokens or points), and child's response in this situation. Ask two or three parents to share their responses to this exercise.
- Ask parents to submit the A-B-C Worksheets that they completed for homework. Ask one or two parents to share their experiences using the worksheet during the week.
- Address problems that parents are having with the completion of assigned homework. Identify specific obstacles encountered by parents, which may include a lack of time, defiance on the part of the child, and parental ambivalence about delivering high rates of positive reinforcement to a child whom they view as highly inattentive and irresponsible. The following strategies may be useful in addressing some of these issues:

    1. Empathize with parents regarding the challenge of changing the homework behavior of a child with ADHD amidst all of the demands they face in their family and professional lives.
    2. Assist parents in arranging their schedules so that they can devote the time needed to address their child's needs during homework.
    3. Remind parents of the CISS-4 principles, and emphasize, in particular, the im-

portance of providing a 4:1 ratio of positive reinforcement to punishment in responding to their child's behavior.

GOAL 2: DESCRIBE THE IMPORTANCE OF TIME MANAGEMENT AND GOAL SETTING

Children with attention and learning problems often are very inefficient in their use of time. When given work to do, they typically waste time and fail to persist with tasks. Because many parents insist that all of their child's assignments be completed, homework can take a very long time for some of these children. Long periods of homework are very frustrating to the child, the parents, and siblings, resulting in increased child defiance, parenting stress, and parent–child conflict. For these reasons, it is critical that parents take control and place limits on the amount of time their child spends doing homework. Relatedly, parents, with the support of teachers, must set realistic expectations for work completion and accuracy and guide their children in setting reasonable goals for themselves.

- Emphasize once again the importance of reducing time spent on homework and getting more work done within the allotted time. Discuss with parents the advantages to the child and family of getting homework done more efficiently. The advantages include: (1) helping the child to develop effective work habits, (2) reducing the child's frustration, (3) reducing parental frustration and stress, (4) improving the parent–child relationship, (5) enabling the child to have more free time to play, and (6) enabling the parents to have more time to devote to other family matters, including spending time with siblings.

- Explain to parents the benefits of setting realistic goals for homework completion, accuracy, and duration and holding children accountable for these goals. The primary advantage is that children are more likely to succeed, resulting in an improvement in the child's sense of self-efficacy and a reduction of frustration and stress.

- Encourage parents to identify obstacles to placing limits on the amount of time children spend doing work. Most parents are concerned that placing limits on homework time will result in a child's failure to complete assignments. Parents often have irrational beliefs about what will happen if children do not complete homework. It is helpful to identify and challenge these beliefs, which might include the following:

1. *"The teacher will not understand and will penalize my child for incomplete work."* Although some teachers may not understand, most teachers are very willing to collaborate with parents whose children spend excessive amounts of time to do homework. Teachers generally are willing to help parents set time limits for homework and to refrain from penalizing a child for partial completion of homework as long as the child is clearly making an attempt to perform assignments. When a teacher is not understanding, consultation with a professional often is helpful. In the Homework Success Program, the clinician will provide teacher consultation to facilitate this process.

2. *"My child will lower his or her standards for success."* In the initial phases of intervention, standards for success may be reduced. By so doing, children typically

experience more success, and the pressure on the family is reduced. As time proceeds and the child begins to experience success on a consistent basis, standards for performance must be raised, or the child may learn to accept mediocre performance and "settle for less."

3. *"I am not effective as a parent if I allow my child get away with substandard performance."* Some parents may believe that they are incompetent as parents if their child does not achieve 100% rates of homework completion and accuracy. Clinicians need to remind parents that this belief system can result in high rates of failure and a disproportionate amount of punitive as opposed to positive feedback to the child, which is not effective parenting.

GOAL 3: PROVIDE INSTRUCTION IN HOW TO MANAGE TIME AND SET GOALS

Managing time and setting appropriate goals for homework is a challenging task for parents. Parents will need detailed instruction in how to manage time and set goals during homework. The Goal-Setting Tool is an instrument that helps to operationalize the steps of time management and goal setting. Group leaders will need to spend a significant portion of the session on introducing the GST, demonstrating its usage, and assisting parents in learning and practicing the technique.

- Distribute *Handout 13: Managing Time and Goal Setting.*
- Explain that managing time and setting appropriate goals is a challenging task for both parents and children. At the outset, these procedures may seem complicated and difficult; however, our experience is that, with practice, these techniques will make sense and will become easier to use.
- Tell parents that the critical variables for them to focus on when using these procedures are rates of completion, rates of accuracy, and duration or amount of time spent on the assignment. Other variables, such as attention to task, fidgeting, talking, and arguing, are less important and should not be the focus of parents' attention. Emphasize that if the parents can be successful in helping the child to get more work completed and achieve higher rates of accuracy in less time, the child will automatically become more attentive and less disruptive.
- Demonstrate the use of time-management and goal-setting procedures before describing each step of the procedures. There are several ways to do this:

    1. Make a videotape of a parent and child using the goal-setting procedures successfully, and show this to the parents.
    2. Ask one of the children to come into the room and provide a live demonstration to the parents of how to use the procedures.
    3. Role play the use of the procedures with a cofacilitator or parent.

- Describe in a step-by-step fashion the procedures for managing time and setting goals. Refer the parents to *Handout 13: Managing Time and Goal Setting* when providing these instructions.

1. Step 1 is to review the homework assignment book and to segment homework into manageable units. Underscore the fact that segmenting is particularly important for children with ADHD, as it has been shown that these children tend to display deficits in organizing their time and work. Discuss methods of segmenting homework. For example, it is often useful for parents to segment work according to the subjects children are assigned for homework. However, if the child has a great deal of homework in one particular subject, the work may need to be segmented into two or more subunits. For instance, a math homework sheet that contains 20 problems may need to be broken up into two subunits of 10 problems each.

2. Step 2 is to set time limits for each subunit of work. Tell parents that the weekly logs of time spent on homework that they have been keeping will be helpful in estimating how long it should take a child to complete work in a particular subject. A general guideline for subunit length is three times the grade level of the child. Thus a fourth-grade student, for example, may have segments of 10 to 12 minutes apiece. Stress to parents that this is only a guideline and that they may have to adjust the subunit length according to their own experiences. The key is to be generous with time estimates so that the child has a good chance of being successful with a reasonable degree of effort. At this time, group leaders should refer to the sample Goal-Setting Tool and direct parents to the box labeled "Step 1: What is my goal?" The child is to indicate the time to be spent on each subunit in the space labeled *Time.*

3. In Step 3 the parents and child negotiate goals for work completion. Discuss with parents the importance of including the child in the process of establishing goals. At the same time, highlight the idea that children need guidance in setting goals, as they often overestimate what they are able to accomplish. Remind parents to be liberal in their estimations of what the child can reasonably accomplish at this time, particularly while the family is in the initial stages of using this procedure. A long-term goal is for 100% of the work to be completed. However, it is more important at this stage for both the parent and child to experience success with this procedure. Therefore, they may need to set completion goals initially in the 50–80% range. Stress to parents that, in estimating completion goals, the guiding principle should be to design situations so that children can meet goals and experience success 80% of the time. Refer parents to Step 1 of the Goal-Setting Tool, in which the number of items completed is indicated.

4. Step 4 is to negotiate with the child to set reasonable accuracy goals. Once again, emphasize to parents that they need to establish accuracy goals that will ensure that the child meets goals and experiences success at least 80% of the time. Parents should refer to their daily logs in assisting the child to establish reasonable goals for accuracy. Refer parents to Step 1 of the Goal-Setting Tool, in which the number of items correct is indicated.

5. Step 5 is to look over the assignment and make sure that the child understands the directions and how to complete the task. At this point, it is appro-

priate for the parent to offer assistance to the child. The parent may wish to demonstrate how to complete a problem and to provide guidance when the child works on a problem. The parent should provide tutoring in this manner until it is clear that the child knows what to do. Then the parent should shift from being the child's homework tutor to being the supervisor.

6. In Step 6 the child starts working on a subunit of homework. Parents are encouraged to use a countdown timer to ensure that time limits are followed.

7. In Step 7 parents should remain close enough to the child to carefully observe and to provide praise when the child is being productive. Help parents to understand that it is important to provide praise frequently, although not so often that it becomes a distraction. Providing praise every 1 to 2 minutes is a good rule of thumb. Emphasize the importance of ignoring inattentive, attention-seeking behavior. About midway through the time period, a parent can approach the child to see if he or she needs help. The parent can provide help briefly but should not interact with the child for more than a half minute or so. If the child asks for help during the time period, the parent should tell the child to wait until the midpoint or endpoint of the time period for this subunit.

8. Step 8 pertains to the evaluation of the child's performance. At the end of the time limit, the parent and the child look over the work and determine rates of work completion and accuracy. Parents should encourage the child to count the number of items completed. Parents can then assist the child in determining the number of items performed correctly. The child should enter the data pertaining to work completion and accuracy in the box labeled "Step 2: How Did I Do?" in the Goal-Setting Tool. In all likelihood, some of the work will be completed inaccurately. Although incorrect items are noted, no additional time is spent going over this subunit of work. If the child chooses to go over the work later, on his or her own time, this is permissible. However, it is important that the parent not spend any additional time working with the child on subunits of work that have already been covered.

9. In Step 9, the parents and child need to evaluate whether goals have been achieved. There are three possibilities: "did not meet goal"; "met goal"; and "exceeded goal." These ratings can readily be used to determine points earned in a token reinforcement system. For example, "did not meet goal" = 0 points; "met goal" = 1 point; and "exceeded goal" = 2 points. Children can earn points for both work completion and work accuracy.

10. Step 10 is to move on to the next subunit of homework and to follow the goal-setting procedure, using Steps 1 through 9.

- Model for the parents once again how to use time-management and goal-setting procedures. Ideally, the clinician can model the use of these procedures by working with a child, but if this is not possible, a role play with a cofacilitator or parent can be arranged.

- Request that the parents practice the time-management and goal-setting procedures using the Goal-Setting Tool. Once again, it is ideal for the parents to practice with their own child, but if this is not possible, the parents can break into dyads and practice with each other. The clinician should observe each of the parents using the goal-setting strategies and provide feedback to them.

• Emphasize once again that the goal-setting strategy can seem complicated and burdensome in the beginning but that over time and with practice parents typically are comfortable using the procedures and can see the effects of the technique.

HOMEWORK ASSIGNMENTS FOR PARENTS

The following are the homework assignments for this session. Make sure that the parents write down the assignments on the Weekly Family Assignment Sheet.

• Request that the parents explain the time-management and goal-setting procedures to their child. The technique can sound very complicated, so it is important for the parents to provide a brief description to the child.

• Request that the parents use the Goal-Setting Tool with each subunit of work. Ask the parents to save the data and to submit it at the following session.

• Ask the parents to meet with the teacher during the week. At this meeting the parents should:

1. Thank the teacher for contributing to the child's progress with homework.
2. Solicit the teacher's feedback about homework performance.
3. Inform the teacher about the time-management and goal-setting procedures being used. Explain to the teacher that the child may continue to submit work that is incomplete and somewhat inaccurate during the early stages of implementing the goal-setting procedures.
4. Inform the teacher about goals for work completion in each subject. Negotiate with him or her a method for evaluating work that is incomplete and inaccurate during the initial stages of implementing the goal-setting intervention.
5. Negotiate a method of parent–teacher communication that keeps the teacher informed about changes in goals for homework completion and accuracy.

• Ask the parents to continue using the A-B-C Worksheet when problems arise during homework. Ask the parents to complete this worksheet at least two times in the coming week.

CLINICIAN CONSULTATION WITH THE TEACHER

After this session, clinicians are encouraged to consult with teachers. If possible, the clinician should arrange to be present when the parents meet with the teacher after Session 4. If this is not feasible, which is often the case when Homework Success is offered in a clinic setting, then clinicians can provide the consultation by phone. The clinician should do the following things during the consultation:

- Request feedback from the teacher about the child's progress with homework.
- Thank the teacher for using the homework assignment book and continuing to complete outcome measures.
- Explain the purpose of limiting time spent on homework and setting reasonable goals for completion and accuracy.
- Inform the teacher about the time-management and goal-setting strategies being used. Solicit the teacher's ideas about how to refine these procedures.
- Explain that the short-term consequence of using these procedures is that the child may complete less work or work less accurately. Negotiate with the teacher a strategy for addressing these concerns.
- Obtain outcome data from the teacher. Specifically, ask the teacher to complete the Academic Performance Rating Scale, submit samples of the child's homework and classwork, and submit copies of records of homework, classwork, and test performance.

CHAPTER 11

Group Session 5:
Using Punishment Successfully

GOALS

1. Review homework.
2. Refine skills in goal setting and time management.
3. Educate parents about punishment.
4. Train parents to use punishment strategically.

This session focuses on helping parents to reflect on the value of punishment, to understand its effects and side effects, and to learn the importance of using punishment in the context of a system that utilizes primarily positive reinforcement methods. Many parents enter intervention programs such Homework Success using punishment too frequently and using methods of punishment that are not effective. This session is designed to educate parents about methods of punishment that can be effective and to assist parents in delivering punishment in a way that will be successful. To prepare for this session, group leaders should have the following materials:

- The integrity checklist that corresponds with Session 5 (Appendix C).
- The following handouts (Appendix D):
  Handout 14: Goal Setting Tool: Summary Worksheet
  Handout 15: Using Punishment Successfully

GOAL 1: REVIEW HOMEWORK

Because the parents were given some very challenging homework assignments to perform, group leaders may need to spend a considerable amount of time reviewing assignments. In addition to reviewing homework assigned at the previous session, clinicians are encouraged to assess parents' progress in implementing previously learned skills, such as using the homework ritual, giving effective commands, and using positive reinforcement.

- Ask parents to submit their weekly logs of homework completion, accuracy, and duration.
- Ask parents to share their child's homework assignment book and provide feedback.
- Discuss with parents their experiences in explaining the Goal-Setting Tool to their children. Identify techniques the parents used to facilitate a dialogue with their child, and offer praise.
- Review the implementation of the Goal-Setting Tool. Elicit feedback about successes and problems. Encourage parents to discuss their concerns about this procedure with the group. Parents will often express concern about work that is not completed after time limits have expired. Group leaders need to emphasize that parents are not to help children with a subunit of homework after the time limit for that unit has expired. Also, parents will often remark that the Goal-Setting Tool seems very time-consuming and unnatural. It is important to empathize with the parents and to remind them that this technique can be very helpful if they persist and gain more practice using it.
- Collect the Goal-Setting Tool worksheet completed by the parents and provide feedback.
- Discuss with the parents the meeting they had with their child's teacher. Ask parents to report on the discussion they had with the teacher about how to evaluate homework that has not been completed. Also, ask parents if they were able to work out a mechanism to communicate with the teacher about changes in goals for work completion and accuracy as they occur in the future.
- Discuss with parents the consultation you had with the teacher. Identify and address issues in home–school communication that still need to be addressed.
- Ask parents to submit their A-B-C Worksheets. Encourage at least one set of parents to share their analysis with the group.

GOAL 2: REFINE SKILLS IN GOAL SETTING AND TIME MANAGEMENT

It is important that parents continue to practice the steps of the Goal-Setting Tool, so that the skills of goal setting and time management become further developed and more effectively implemented for each homework assignment. Parents will be provided with a summary version of the Goal-Setting Tool that is easier to implement once this technique is fully learned.

- Distribute the Goal-Setting Tool to parents once again and review the steps of this intervention. Encourage parents to ask specific questions about this technique now that they have had a week to use it.
- Distribute *Handout 14: Goal Setting Tool: Summary Worksheet*. Explain to parents

that these summary worksheets will enable the family to record data from several sub-units of work on the same page. Make sure the parents understand how to use the worksheets and provide an illustration. Encourage parents to use the summary worksheets once they are competent with the basic goal-setting steps.

GOAL 3: EDUCATE PARENTS ABOUT PUNISHMENT

For punishment to be effective, it must be implemented strategically. Punishment should be delivered in a well-planned manner in response to specifically targeted, problematic behaviors. Parents should select a method of punishment that can be effective with minimal side effects and that is embedded within the context of a positive reinforcement system. Thus parents need to understand the purposes of punishment and the adverse effects associated with these consequences.

- Distribute *Handout 15: Using Punishment Successfully.*
- Describe the rationale for using punishment as a strategy to change children's behavior. Highlight the following points:

  1. Whereas positive reinforcement is primarily useful in promoting skill development and increasing desirable behaviors, punishment is often helpful in the reduction of problem behaviors.
  2. Positive reinforcement methods may not be sufficient to change targeted behaviors, especially for children who have ADHD.
  3. The strategic use of punishment can enhance the contrast between the consequences for adaptive versus nonadaptive behavior, thus leading to a more rapid change in behavior.

- Describe the potential adverse effects of using punishment, including:

  1. Punishment generally fails to teach new skills or to increase the frequency of adaptive behaviors.
  2. Punishment may increase a child's oppositional, defiant behaviors.
  3. Punishment may increase the conflict between parents and their child.
  4. Punishment, particularly when delivered in a harsh, aggressive manner, may lead the child to behave aggressively.

GOAL 4: TRAIN PARENTS TO USE PUNISHMENT STRATEGICALLY

To be effective, punishment must be delivered within the context of a primarily positive system of reinforcement. Specific behaviors should be targeted for change. Parents need to be firm and under control emotionally when delivering punishment. Also, parents should understand that there are two types of punishment: removing positive reinforcement and administering mildly aversive consequences. Two types of punishment that can be successful if implemented properly are response cost and correction. Corporal punishment is not recommended under any circumstances. Time-out is recommended only in rare cases for homework problems because this consequence often provides reinforcement for avoiding work. In discussing methods of punishment, parents need to be reminded of the CISS-4 principles.

- Inform parents that punishment is most effective when it is delivered in response to specific behaviors that have been targeted for change. Appropriate target behaviors for punishment are those that are highly problematic and occur relatively infrequently (e.g., hitting a sibling, cursing at a parent, throwing an object). In addition, punishment can be used with high-frequency behaviors (e.g., getting out of his or her seat, talking to a sibling), but it is critical that parents target only one or two high-frequency behaviors so that punishment is not used too often. We strongly recommend that parents use positive reinforcement methods and not punishment to address problems with attention and productivity, particularly at the outset. Encourage parents to identify one or two homework behaviors that would be appropriate targets for punishment.

- Emphasize that parents need to be firm and in control emotionally when administering punishment to their child. Discuss with parents the importance of monitoring their emotional responses to their child's misbehavior. When parents become frustrated and angry, it is often difficult for them to maintain emotional control when delivering punishment. Encourage parents to share their emotional reactions to the misbehavior that occurs during homework. Also, ask parents how they deal with their emotions and how they actually administer punishment. Help them to understand the link between emotions and behavior. Most parents overreact when their child's behavior is highly problematic. Encourage parents to discuss methods they have used to control their emotions when responding to their child. Identify useful strategies for controlling emotional responses and praise parents for their efforts to control their emotions in delivering punishment.

- Remind parents of the CISS-4 principles. Review each of the principles (consistency, immediacy, specificity, saliency, and 4:1 ratio) and discuss the importance of using positive reinforcers at least four times more often than punishers.

- Inform parents about the two types of punishment: removing positive reinforcement and administering mildly aversive consequences. Tell them that the removal of positive reinforcement is an underused method of punishment that can be highly effective when used correctly.

- Provide examples of how to remove positive reinforcement:

    1. *Response cost.* Explain to parents that response cost refers to the removal of a positive reinforcer in response to an inappropriate behavior. Provide examples of response cost. Turning off the television when a child hits a sibling is an example of response cost. Also, if the family is using a token reinforcement system, taking a token away from the child in response to a targeted misbehavior is a response-cost intervention. Discuss with parents how they can incorporate a response-cost component into their token reinforcement system.

    2. *Time-out.* Explain to parents that time-out refers to the systematic removal of as many things that are positively reinforcing to a child as possible. Typically, time-out involves placement of a child in a quiet, nonstimulating area of the

house where the child cannot readily gain access to positive reinforcers such as parent and sibling attention, watching TV, and playing with toys. Explain that time-out is only effective if it results in a significant loss of positive reinforcement delivered to the child. A problem with using time-out during homework is that it may provide the child with an opportunity to avoid work demands. In this case, time-out does not result in a reduction of reinforcement. In fact, time-out may actually provide reinforcement to the child, as it enables him or her to gain access to a situation that is more desirable than persisting with a challenging task. For this reason, we rarely recommend using time-out as a strategy to cope with problems during homework.

• Provide examples of how to deliver mild aversive consequences. The only type of mild aversive consequence that we recommend using is *correction*, which can be delivered verbally and nonverbally. Under no circumstance do we recommend corporal punishment, because of the possibility that it will further damage the parent–child relationship and aggravate the child's behavior problems. Provide the following guidelines for delivering correction:

1. State the correction briefly and clearly.
2. Be firm in offering correction and make sure that your emotions are under control.
3. Make sure that your actions match your words when offering correction. For example, when correcting your child, do not smile or laugh.
4. Refrain from making sarcastic comments. For example, comments such as, "It's about time you did some work," will only antagonize the child and may be counterproductive.
5. When correcting a child, state what the child should be doing and do not focus on what the child is not doing. For example, it is much better to say, "Pay attention to your work," as opposed to, "You are not paying attention to work."
6. Comment on a specific aspect of the child's behavior and do not make reference to presumed personality traits of the child. For example, it is better to say, "You need to read the directions more carefully" than to say, "Why do you have to be so lazy?"
7. After offering correction, observe the child carefully, note when the child exhibits behavior that reflects compliance with your correction, and offer praise.

HOMEWORK ASSIGNMENTS FOR PARENTS

Administer the following homework assignments after this session:

• Request that the parents begin using the Goal-Setting Tool: Summary Worksheets each day during homework.
• Request that the parents discuss with their child appropriate methods of punish-

ment. In particular, ask the parents to negotiate with the child a fair way to use response cost as part of their token reinforcement system.

- Ask the parents to speak with their child and to identify one or two behaviors that occur during homework that will be targeted for punishment.

- Ask the parents to complete the A-B-C Worksheet on at least three occasions when they used response cost or correction in response to their child's unproductive or irresponsible behavior.

- Remind the parents of the CISS-4 principles and tell them to make sure they are providing positive reinforcement at least four times more often than punishment.

- Remind the parents to continue filling out the daily parent logs of homework completion, accuracy, and efficiency.

- Remind the parents that the following week's session is the last one of the series of six. Encourage them to work on integrating all of the skills they have developed in the program.

## CHAPTER 12

Group Session 6: Integrating Skills and Anticipating Future Problems

---

GOALS

1. Review homework.
2. Summarize progress and identify continuing problems.
3. Review Homework Success strategies.
4. Develop individualized homework plans.
5. Obtain outcome data.

The purposes of this session are to review the strategies introduced in this program, to provide parents with an opportunity to troubleshoot problems that persist or can be anticipated, and to consolidate the skills acquired during the course of the program. To prepare for the future, participants receive guidance in identifying problems that are particularly challenging for them and in developing a plan to address these concerns. During the session, parents are encouraged to develop an individualized "formula for success" that includes the combination of strategies and techniques that they have found particularly helpful in addressing their child's problems with homework. At the end of the session, time is allotted to celebrate the progress families have made through their participation in Homework Success. Clinicians should prepare for this session by having the following materials available:

- The integrity checklist that corresponds with Session 6 (Appendix C).
- *Handout 16: Maintaining Success and Anticipating Future Problems* (Appendix D).
- The following outcome measures (Appendix B):
  Homework Performance Questionnaire
  Conflict Behavior Questionnaire–Parent and Child Versions
  Homework Success Evaluation Inventory

GOAL 1: REVIEW HOMEWORK

As before, begin each session with a review of homework assigned at the previous session. The parents have many assignments due for this session, but hopefully by this point they have acquired good habits as far as completing their work.

- Ask parents to submit the daily logs of homework completion, accuracy, and duration.
- Ask parents to share with group leaders their child's homework assignment book.
- Request that parents submit the Goal-Setting Tool: Summary Worksheets they completed during the previous week. Encourage parents to discuss their experiences using these worksheets. Identify problems with implementation and provide specific suggestions for addressing each concern. Praise parents for using this intervention each day and for being conscientious in the application of the technique.
- Ask parents to report on the conversation they had with their child about appropriate methods of punishment. Encourage parents to talk about how they and their child decided to incorporate response-cost procedures into their token reinforcement system.
- Ask parents to report the homework behaviors that they targeted for punishment.
- Ask parents to submit the A-B-C Worksheets they completed during the week. Encourage one or two parents to share the analysis they conducted on an occasion when they provided punishment to their child during homework.

GOAL 2: SUMMARIZE PROGRESS AND IDENTIFY CONTINUING PROBLEMS

Parents are encouraged to examine their progress in addressing their child's problems with homework. In doing so, some parents will express concern that they have not addressed all of their child's problems. Parents need to identify problems that have not yet been addressed so that a plan can be developed to address these ongoing concerns.

- Request that parents complete the Homework Performance Questionnaire.
- Share with parents a copy of the Homework Performance Questionnaire that they completed at baseline. Ask parents to note differences between baseline and current performance. Praise parents for their accomplishments. At the same time, note problems that persist. Engage the group in a discussion about how to modify procedures to address persisting problems.

GOAL 3: REVIEW HOMEWORK SUCCESS STRATEGIES

During this session parents review each of the strategies presented during the program. As each strategy is discussed, parents will evaluate their success with implementation.

This activity gives parents the opportunity to identify the strategies they have mastered and have found most acceptable. Also, parents may identify techniques that should be further refined.

- Distribute *Handout 16: Maintaining Success and Anticipating Future Problems.*
- Review the core elements of each session and encourage parents to evaluate the extent to which each approach has been effective in helping their child. Review each of the following components.

1. *ADHD and homework.* At this point in training, parents should have a much better understanding of the relationship between ADHD and homework-related behaviors. Ask parents to express their thoughts about how ADHD has contributed to the problems they and their child have had with homework. Emphasize that a better understanding of their child's and their own limitations helps to avoid the tendency to assign blame when problems arise.

2. *The homework ritual.* Review the "when, where, and what" of homework. Remind parents of the importance of establishing a context for homework that is conducive to being attentive and productive. Ask parents to comment about changes they have made in their child's homework ritual. Assist parents who have found it difficult to adhere to a consistent homework ritual.

3. *Effective instructions.* Ask parents to discuss changes they have made in giving instructions to their child. Emphasize the importance of being brief, clear, and specific in giving directions. Stress that being effective in giving instructions is a prerequisite to increasing compliance. As parents volunteer changes they have made in giving instructions, praise the effective elements and offer suggestions for how to refine their use of the strategy.

4. *Positive reinforcement.* Review the principle of positive reinforcement and remind parents of the importance of using positive reinforcement to change their child's behavior. Review the basic elements of a token reinforcement system, with particular emphasis on identifying targets for intervention, establishing a reward menu, determining points earned for performing each target behavior, and determining how many points each reinforcer is worth. Ask parents to describe the system they are currently using and identify elements of their systems that need to be refined. Also, review the CISS-4 principles with the parents.

5. *Time management and goal setting.* Ask parents to discuss their experiences using the Goal-Setting Tool. Many parents will report that this technique has enabled their child to become more productive and efficient in completing homework. However, some parents may continue to struggle with this procedure. Praise parents for their success and provide suggestions for how to refine their use of this technique.

6. *Punishment.* Review the principle of punishment and remind parents of the importance of using this technique properly. Because parents have been focusing on how to deliver punishment during the previous week and during the homework review, group leaders may not need to spend much time re-

viewing this procedure. Stress, once again, the importance of administering positive reinforcement at least four times more frequently than punishment.

GOAL 4: DEVELOP INDIVIDUALIZED HOMEWORK PLANS

At this point in the session, parents are provided an opportunity to develop their own formula for success, consisting of strategies that they have found to be particularly useful in addressing their child's problems with homework. Parents are encouraged to consolidate what they have learned and to personalize the program. Each participant's formula for success will include the techniques that they have found to be particularly helpful, variations in the strategies that have worked for them, and helpful reminders that will enable them to implement the techniques accurately and consistently in the future.

- Ask each participant to identify the strategies that they have found to be most successful in addressing their child's homework problems. Encourage parents to write the strategies on a notepad.
- Ask the parents to share any adaptations they made in the strategies to enable them to be more effective in helping their child.
- Assist the parents in identifying reminders and tips that will help them to implement strategies in the most effective way.
- Ask the parents to write out their formula for success. For example, the formula might be: Start work at 4:00 P.M. at the kitchen table + make sure to turn off the TV in the next room + apply the Goal-Setting Tool + use a token reinforcement system + make sure to allow enough time in the evening to play a game if the child earns enough points + do not yell at the child during homework.
- Urge parents to have a discussion with their child about their formula for success. The formula that is derived mutually by the parents and child should be posted in a place where they can refer to it as needed. When their child is having a bad day with homework, the parents should refer to their formula for success and make sure they are closely following it.
- Explain to parents that this is the last of the series of six weekly sessions. Inform them that a booster session will be scheduled in about 4 weeks. The purpose of this session is to review their progress, identify problems that have arisen, and further develop strategies to address these concerns.

GOAL 5: OBTAIN OUTCOME DATA

Given that this is the last of the weekly sessions, it is important to collect outcome data from parents. Parents have been providing data on an ongoing basis by submitting the daily logs of homework completion, accuracy, and duration and by completing the Homework Performance Questionnaire periodically. This is a good time to obtain outcome data pertaining to family functioning, intervention acceptability, and program satisfaction.

- Administer the Conflict Behavior Questionnaire—Parent Version and ask parents to complete it.
- Distribute the Conflict Behavior Questionnaire—Child version. If there is a child group, children can complete this measure in their group. If not, parents can ask their child to complete this measure and mail it back. Given the nature of the questions on this checklist, the child's responses are more likely to be accurate if the child completes the form privately.
- Administer the Homework Success Evaluation Inventory and ask parents to complete it.
- Inform parents that you will be contacting the teacher to obtain additional outcome data.

HOMEWORK ASSIGNMENTS FOR PARENTS

- Ask the parents to collaborate with their child to develop their formula for success. Ask them to write down the formula and to post it in a prominent location in the home.
- Encourage the parents to continue using the A-B-C Worksheets whenever a problem arises during homework.
- Encourage the parents to review all of the Homework Success handouts as a way of helping them to refine the ways in which they apply each technique.
- Request that parents schedule a follow-up meeting with their child's teacher. The purposes of this meeting are to (1) review the child's progress with homework and overall academic functioning, (2) identify areas of improvement, (3) identify areas that are still in need of intervention, (4) modify homework interventions to address persisting problems, and (5) thank the teacher for working with them on the Homework Success Program.
- Schedule the booster session.

ARRANGING FOR A CELEBRATION

Families have invested an enormous amount of time and energy in participating in Homework Success. Allow about 15 minutes at the end of the session to acknowledge their accomplishments and to celebrate the progress they have made. If a child group is meeting concurrently, bring the children and parents together for the celebration. We recommend that food be served during the celebration.

OBTAINING OUTCOME DATA FROM THE TEACHER

After this session, contact the teacher and make arrangements to collect outcome data. Specifically, ask the teacher to complete the Academic Performance Rating Scale, submit samples of the child's homework and classwork, and submit copies of records of homework, classwork, and test performance. If the teacher is busy and will have trouble compiling these materials, offer assistance with photocopying, if appropriate. Also, inform the teacher that parents have completed the core sessions of Homework Success. Ask the teacher to comment on the child's progress and to identify problems that still need to be addressed. Thank the teacher for investing in the program and supporting the parents.

## CHAPTER 13

Group Session 7:
Providing Follow-Up Support

GOALS

1. Review progress.
2. Review core components of Homework Success.
3. Identify problems and modify intervention plans.
4. Provide resources to parents.
5. Collect program evaluation data and congratulate parents.

The purpose of this session is to review with parents the progress they have made with homework over the past several weeks. Most parents have encountered some success, as well as some problems. Successes should be acknowledged and reinforced; problems should be identified and plans developed to address each of them. At the previous session, parents were asked to develop a formula for success. During this session, parents should be asked to evaluate this formula and to make any modifications needed to ensure success in the future. This is the final scheduled meeting of the program; therefore, parents need to anticipate the problems that might arise in the future and to develop a plan for how to address these concerns when they arise. At the conclusion of this session, parents are in a good position to evaluate the program and to offer useful feedback to group leaders. Clinicians should prepare for this group by having the following materials available.

- The integrity checklist for Session 7 (Appendix C).
- *Handout 17: Resources* (Appendix D).
- The following outcome measures (Appendix B):
  Homework Performance Questionnaire
  Homework Success Evaluation Inventory
  Homework Success Program Evaluation Scale

GOAL 1: REVIEW PROGRESS

At the outset of this session, clinicians should review with parents the progress they have made in helping their child with homework over the past several weeks. Since the previous session, the parents should have reached an agreement with their child about a formula for success. Also, the parents should have had a meeting with the teacher to review progress.

- Request that parents submit daily logs of homework completion, accuracy, and duration.
- Ask parents to complete the Homework Performance Questionnaire.
- Request that parents share their child's homework assignment book.
- Ask parents to report on their formula for success. Encourage parents to share with the other participants what the formula is, how well they are adhering to it, and how well it works. Note aspects of the formula that are not working well so that these can be addressed later in the session.
- Ask parents to report on the meetings they had with their children's teachers since the previous session. Encourage parents to report on the teachers' views of their children's progress with homework and classwork. Also, request that the parents note problems that persist with school performance.

GOAL 2: REVIEW CORE COMPONENTS OF HOMEWORK SUCCESS

Although parents previously reviewed the core strategies of Homework Success, it is usually helpful to review them again. In particular, parents need reminders that (1) homework is very challenging for inattentive, impulsive children; (2) a consistent homework ritual is important; (3) the A-B-C method is very useful for analyzing problems and planning strategies; (4) positive reinforcement methods are very effective and should be used much more frequently than punishment; (5) setting realistic goals and evaluating performance in relation to these goals is very helpful; and (6) ongoing home–school collaboration is invaluable to homework success.

- Ask parents to refer to *Handout 16: Maintaining Success and Anticipating Future Problems.* This handout reviews the major concepts and strategies contained within Homework Success.
- Review the major concepts and strategies of Homework Success, including:

    1. The relationship between ADHD and homework difficulties.
    2. The homework ritual.
    3. The A-B-C method of assessment.
    4. Giving instructions effectively.
    5. Positive reinforcement and punishment.
    6. Goal setting and time management.
    7. Home–school collaboration.

- Encourage parents to evaluate their effectiveness in using each of these procedures. Request that participants help each other when a parent expresses problems with implementation.

- Stress once again the importance of communicating frequently and effectively with teachers. Emphasize that parents should not be passive and wait for teachers to contact them. Encourage parents to initiate contact with the teacher to learn about homework issues and academic performance. If the teacher expresses a concern, it is important for the parents to arrange a time to meet with the teacher, analyze the situation, and develop a plan.

GOAL 3: IDENTIFY PROBLEMS AND MODIFY INTERVENTION PLANS

Of course, many parents will continue to have problems with some aspects of homework at follow-up. Some parents have become very effective at problem solving when concerns arise, but some will still need guidance. Ask parents to use the A-B-C method to analyze problems and plan interventions.

- Ask each parent to identify current problems they are experiencing with homework.

- Request that they select one problem and conduct an A-B-C analysis of this concern using the Homework A-B-C Worksheet. Also, ask them to generate ideas about an intervention plan based on this analysis.

- Ask each parent to share the results of the analysis, as well as their proposed intervention plan. Encourage the other participants to comment on the analysis and the plan, with particular emphasis on those aspects of the plan that are well designed.

- Ask parents to review their formula for success and to make needed adjustments. Encourage them to go home and have a discussion with their child about their formula for success.

- Stress to parents the importance of using the A-B-C method whenever problems arise in the future.

GOAL 4: PROVIDE RESOURCES TO PARENTS

At this point, most parents realize that homework is an ongoing challenge, particularly for inattentive, impulsive children. Although Homework Success hopefully was helpful for them, there is no magic to this program. Parents need to keep applying the strategies every day and to modify the approaches when needed to be effective. At this point in the session, it is important to discuss resources needed by the parents to ensure success in managing children's homework.

- Distribute *Handout 17: Resources*. Discuss with parents the many resources available to them. Point out that books for parents and children are available to assist them in managing homework and coping with ADHD. Encourage them to contact Children and Adults with ADD (CHADD; 800-233-4050) to learn about local support groups and to obtain additional information.

• Discuss with parents the possibility of scheduling a follow-up booster session within 2 to 3 months. Tell them that most parents find this to be very helpful. If the group decides to arrange a follow-up session, schedule a time for this meeting.

• Inform parents how they can contact you if they have questions or need help coping with homework issues or other matters. Explain that Homework Success is not designed to address all of their family's needs. Many families need additional counseling to address family or school issues or both. Encourage families to call if they need additional help so that appropriate referrals can be made.

GOAL 5: COLLECT PROGRAM EVALUATION DATA AND CONGRATULATE PARENTS

As we discussed previously, collecting outcome data is critical in determining program effectiveness for each child and family and in obtaining suggestions about how to improve the program. These data must be collected from the parents and the teachers.

• Request that parents complete the Homework Success Evaluation Inventory and the Homework Success Program Evaluation Scale.

• As a final exercise, ask each parent to share the one or two things they learned that were the most helpful to them and their family.

• Distribute diplomas to the parents. Congratulate them for their hard work, commitment, and success. Say good-bye and wish them well.

OBTAINING OUTCOME DATA FROM THE TEACHER

After this session, contact the teacher and make arrangements to collect follow-up data. Specifically, ask the teacher to complete the Academic Performance Rating Scale, submit samples of the child's homework and classwork, and submit copies of records of homework, classwork, and test performance. Ask the teacher to comment on the child's progress and to identify problems that still need to be addressed. Thank the teacher for investing in the program and supporting the parents.

CHAPTER 14

Including Children in Homework Success

STEPHEN S. LEFF, JAMES L. KARUSTIS, TRACY E. COSTIGAN,
SUZANNE G. GOLDSTEIN, SHEEBA DANIEL-CROTTY,
DINA F. HABBOUSHE, AND THOMAS J. POWER

A unique feature of the Homework Success Program is that it encourages the involvement of children throughout the process of intervention and includes procedures for coordinating a concurrent child-training group. In contrast, most homework intervention systems include only parents or teachers.

There are a number of reasons why including children in a homework program can further improve homework performance and family functioning. First, student participation in setting goals related to homework accuracy and completion is associated with improvements in homework motivation and performance (Olympia, Sheridan, Jenson, & Andrews, 1994). Second, including both parents and children in treatment allows the intervention to more directly address the parent–child conflicts that can complicate homework procedures and routines (Richters, Arnold, Jensen, & Abikoff, 1995). Third, introducing children to concepts that their parents are learning through parent training has been linked to improvements in the child's understanding and compliance with these interventions (Frankel et al., 1997; Webster-Stratton & Hammond, 1997). For example, group behavioral interventions that include both parent- and child-training components have demonstrated reductions in students' disruptive behaviors and increases in parents' skills in providing positive reinforcement, both immediately following treatment and at 1-year follow-up (Frankel et al., 1997; Kazdin, Siegel, & Bass, 1992; Webster-Stratton & Hammond, 1997). Further, several studies have found that combined parent- and child-training components are more effective than either the parent- or child-training components administered alone (Kazdin et al., 1992; Webster-Stratton & Hammond, 1997). Finally, many of the child participants have found the group to be an informative and extremely enjoyable experience. Thus, there are many advantages to providing a combined child- and parent-training group whenever it is possible.

In this chapter we present an overview of the child-training component of the program, session-by-session guidelines, obstacles to providing this type of child-training program, and recommendations for overcoming obstacles and successfully administering the program. Appendix E contains three handouts that can be used to implement the sessions more successfully.

OVERVIEW OF THE CHILD COMPONENT OF THE HOMEWORK SUCCESS PROGRAM

As described in earlier chapters, Homework Success targets children in grades 1 through 6 who have significant homework difficulties and problems related to ADHD. A trained professional facilitates the child group, and the session topics parallel those covered in the concurrent parent group.

Each session lasts for approximately 1½ hours. The first 15 minutes of each session is devoted to a check-in time that combines child and parent participants. During this time, homework assignments are reviewed, and the current session's goals are introduced. The children and their group leader then move to a separate room to begin their session. As outlined in Table 14.1, each session of the child group follows a highly structured format that includes (1) a joint discussion with the parent group, (2) a review of the group rules and in-session behavior management system, (3) a structured activity, (4) a short break, (5) a second structured activity, and (6) an evaluation of each child's behavior during the session, including the provision of tangible reinforcers based on each child's point total for the session.

The use of behavior management techniques during each session is a critical component of the child group. Given that all participating children have problems related to ADHD and thus are likely to be inattentive and/or hyperactive–impulsive, it is extremely important from the outset to establish a clear and consistent behavior management protocol. Every 15 minutes, the activity is paused to give children feedback about their behavior. For instance, each child can earn between 0 and 2 points for following the established group rules during the preceding 15 minutes. At the end of each session, children exchange their earned points for reinforcers of varying value. Points are not saved from one week to the next week. In addition to facilitating cooperative and compliant behavior within the group, this system orients children to a token reinforcement system that will be instituted at home during the program. Also, valuable clinical information can be provided to parents (and teachers) about how to implement a token reinforcement system with each individual.

To ensure consistency in the delivery of the child component of the Homework Success Program, as with the parent group, it is strongly recommended that the group leader throughout each session utilize an integrity checklist (see Appendix C for an ex-

TABLE 14.1. Homework Success Program: Organization of the Child Group

Time (minutes)	Typical activity	Goals
Every session		
0:00–0:15	Discussion with parent group	• Coordinate parent and child groups. • Review homework assignments. • Introduce current week's topic.
0:15–0:25	Review group rules and behavior management system	• Review group rules and expectations. • Review the in-session token reinforcement system.
0:25–0:45	Structured activity I	• Introduce new topic in a developmentally appropriate format. • Reinforce topic addressed in concurrent parent group.
0:45–0:55	Break	
0:55–1:15	Structured activity II	• Introduce new topic in a developmentally appropriate format. • Reinforce topic addressed in concurrent parent group.
1:15–1:30	Point totals and cash-in	• Provide tangible reinforcement based on child's point total.
Additional component		
0:55–1:05	Weeks 2, 4, 6, and follow-up Administration of acceptability measures	• Evaluate acceptability of child treatment component.

Note. Every 15 minutes, activities are paused and points are reviewed and given as appropriate for each child.

ample of an integrity checklist). This checklist can serve to prompt the group leader to address critical components of each session and to ensure that all group goals and activities are accomplished during each session. As discussed in earlier chapters, treatment acceptability is also a critical aspect in the ongoing implementation of any treatment program. Thus it is recommended that a child report measure, such as the Children's Intervention Rating Profile (Witt & Elliot, 1985), be administered during Sessions 2, 4, and 6 and at the booster session. This 7-item rating scale, modified to specifically evaluate the child component of Homework Success, is a commonly utilized measure that assesses children's opinions about the acceptability of an intervention. The Children's Intervention Rating Profile for the Homework Success Program can be found in Appendix E.

SESSION 1: INTRODUCING HOMEWORK SUCCESS

> **GOALS**
>
> 1. Orient children to the components of the program.
> 2. Define rules and expectations for the group, including use of a token reinforcement system.
> 3. Begin to build group cohesion.
> 4. Discuss homework successes and problems.
> 5. Describe the importance of group homework assignments.

This session is primarily designed to help children understand the main components of Homework Success and the specific rules and expectations for the group. In addition, children are encouraged to begin talking with other children in the group about their own successes and difficulties with homework. Clinicians should prepare for this session by having the following materials available:

- *Supplies.* Two poster-sized pieces of paper for rules and agenda, name tags, prizes, several bags of M&M's candy, concentration cards (question and picture cards), "mystery" prize for the winner of the concentration game, snacks.
- *An integrity checklist for Session 1 (see Appendix C for an example).* The integrity checklists outline the steps to follow during each session. These checklists can prompt clinicians to address the content and process issues pertaining to each session. Clinicians should check each item on the checklist after it has been completed.

Goal 1: Orient Children to the Components of the Program

- After children attend the brief general orientation to the program offered to them and their parents, escort children into the child therapy room.
- Introduce yourself to the group. Briefly describe your interest in working with children who have problems with attention and homework.
- Discuss the purpose of the homework group, highlighting the following points:

  1. Many children have problems with homework. These problems can include difficulties with completing homework, answering homework questions correctly, or remembering to turn in homework to teachers.
  2. Homework difficulties can be stressful for children and families.
  3. The purpose of this group is to talk about these difficulties and to help children find ways to make homework more manageable and enjoyable.
  4. The group is a safe place for discussing feelings related to homework. It is a time for both fun and serious work.

- Review with the children the agenda for the session.

Goal 2: Define Rules and Expectations for the Group, Including Use of a Token Reinforcement System

- Facilitate a discussion of group rules. Guide the conversation so as to ensure that session rules are stated clearly. Make sure that there are only three to four rules and that each rule is stated in a positive manner (e.g., be kind and respectful to others, keep hands and feet to yourself, use appropriate language). As this discussion occurs, write the group rules on a large piece of paper for the entire group to view. The following points should be highlighted:

  1. The purpose of the group rules is to ensure that everyone feels safe and comfortable in the group.
  2. Everyone in the group, group leader and children alike, will develop the rules together.
  3. The rules that the children generate are subject to the group leader's approval.

- Explain the token reinforcement system used in each session (including a discussion about how to earn points). The explanation should include the following points:

  1. Every 15 minutes the group leaders will rate each child on how well they followed each of the rules.
  2. The children earn 0 points if they had difficulty following all or most rules, 1 point if they followed most group rules, 2 points if they followed all group rules well.
  3. Children are *not* allowed to contest the number of points they receive. If children protest, they should be reminded that the points are not negotiable and that they can try harder to get 2 points at the next checkpoint.
  4. The number of points children receive at each checkpoint are independent of their previous points. This means that regardless of how few or how many points a child earned at the first checkpoint, he or she has the opportunity to earn up to 2 points at the next checkpoint.
  5. At the end of the session, the children will be allowed to choose a reward based on the number of total points they have received throughout the session. Small (i.e., stickers), medium (i.e., pencils), and large (i.e., small toys) prizes should be given based on how many total points a child has received. The number of points needed for each level of the prizes should be determined at the first session and can be changed in later sessions if indicated. The token system should be set up so that the majority of children receive medium or large prizes and so that all of the children earn rewards.
  6. At this time child participants should be asked if they have any questions.
  7. After questions are finished, the group leader tells the children that the token reinforcement system will begin.

Goal 3: Begin to Build Group Cohesion

- Introduce the *Getting-to-Know-You Game* This brief game is utilized to help children feel more comfortable in the group, to facilitate discussion, and to normalize the problems that participants may be experiencing.

- Provide instructions for the *Getting-To-Know-You Game.* Have everyone sit in a circle. Pass around a bag of M&M's candy and ask each child to take up to five M&M's. Next, ask each child to say one thing about himself or herself for each M&M that they are holding. Each time they say something about themselves, they can eat one of the M&M's.

- Provide children with examples of the kinds of things they can discuss (e.g., school, grades, siblings, favorite activities, hobbies). Children should be made to feel safe and comfortable. Some children may need assistance in articulating their responses. In this instance, ask the child specific questions (e.g., What is your name? What school do you go to? Do you have any brothers or sisters?).

- Take a 5-minute break. In order to minimize any difficulties the children may have with transitions, it is important to explain what will be occurring during the break and what is expected during this time. Explain that the group will be taking a short break, during which time each child will be given a snack and will have opportunities to talk with others and to use the bathroom. Remind children that they must continue to follow all group rules during the break. Tell the children that they will be asked to sit down quietly and listen to the group leader explain the next activity following the break.

Goal 4: Discuss Homework Successes and Problems

- Introduce the *Homework Questions Concentration Game.* This game allows children to begin to express their thoughts and feelings regarding homework in an enjoyable and structured manner. Sample game cards are provided in Appendix E.

- Provide instructions for the Homework Questions Concentration Game. Instruct children to sit in a circle while you place the homework concentration cards face down in a square grid. The children should be told that each child will get a turn as they go around in a circle. Each child should be instructed to choose two cards and informed that the goal is to try to choose two picture cards that are identical to each other or to choose a card with a question on it. If a child gets a card with a question on it, he or she answers the question. Then the other children answer the same question. If the child who chose the question card provides an adequate answer to the question, he or she gets to keep it, and it counts for 1 point. If a child gets two matching pictures, he or she gets to keep the cards, and they count for 1 point. If a child gets two picture cards that do not match, he or she places the cards back, and the turn passes to the next child. Whoever has the most points at the end of the game wins the game and receives a small "mystery" prize.

- Include the following questions in the Homework Questions Concentration Game:

  1. Name one problem you have when you do your homework.
  2. What do you think your parents find hard about your homework?
  3. Name one thing your parents can do to make your homework easier.
  4. Name one thing you can do to make homework easier for yourself.
  5. How can you make your homework fun?

- Provide frequent verbal praise for cooperation. Emphasize that children should enjoy the game and discuss the questions as opposed to competing with other children.

Goal 5: Describe the Importance of Group Homework Assignments

- Inform the children that their parents will be completing homework assignments between each session and that many times the children will also be included in these assignments. Between Sessions 1 and 2 the parents will be assigned a number of specific activities.
- Let the children know that their parents have been asked to sit down with them to discuss what homework is like for each of them, including a discussion of why homework is important and how frustrating their problems with homework can be for the entire family.
- Inform the children that one of the first things they will notice is that there is now a time limit for completing their homework and that they should try to get as much homework completed as possible during this time. However, stress the importance of working carefully on assignments.
- Introduce the A-B-C logs (Appendix B). It is not important to discuss the specifics of these logs. Merely mention that the parents have been asked to keep track of the child's homework each day, including each child's behavior during homework time. A-B-C logs are a helpful tool for making homework proceed smoothly and are used throughout the program.

Conclusion of Session 1

Session 1 and all other sessions should be concluded with the following activities:

- Tell each child the total number of points that he or she earned throughout the session. Instruct the child to choose a prize (small, medium, or large) based on the number of total points earned.
- Emphasize positive behaviors displayed by each child in the session. Do not focus excessively on disruptive behaviors but simply exhort the children to keep up the good effort throughout the week and into the next session.
- End the group by reviewing the session's activities. For instance, it is important to review the rules established for the group and to summarize children's main comments in regard to their homework successes and difficulties.

SESSION 2: ESTABLISHING A HOMEWORK RITUAL AND GIVING INSTRUCTIONS

> **GOALS**
>
> 1. Review group homework assignments.
> 2. Review group rules and token reinforcement system.
> 3. Continue to build group cohesion.
> 4. Help children to improve their homework routines and to identify potential reinforcers.
> 5. Discuss group homework assignments.

This session is designed to help children better understand and improve their homework routines. By the end of the session, they should be able to identify an appropriate place within the home to complete homework, the materials needed to begin homework, and reinforcers they would like to receive for appropriate homework performance. Clinicians should prepare for this session by having the following materials available:

- *Supplies.* Two poster-sized pieces of paper for rules and agenda, name tags, prizes, "mystery" prize for the Fabulous Four Game, cards for the Fabulous Four Game, timer, snacks.
- *An integrity checklist for Session 2.* Clinicians should check each item on the checklist after it has been completed.

Goal 1: Review Group Homework Assignments

- Review the previous session's assignments with the parents and children during the initial 15 minutes of the session.
- Facilitate a discussion about what it was like for parents and children to sit down and talk about the importance of homework and the stressors that it can place on the family.
- Ask parents and children about the time limit that parents placed on homework during the past week.
- Request that the child complete the Children's Intervention Rating Profile (Appendix E).

Goal 2: Review Group Rules and Token Reinforcement System

- Lead children into the child therapy room to begin the session.
- Review the rules and the token reinforcement system.
- Remind children that the reinforcement system is to begin at this point.
- Provide an overview of the session's activities. This could include posting and

then reviewing an agenda of the session's activities with the children. This will help each child learn the typical routine for the group.

Goal 3: Continue to Build Group Cohesion

Building group cohesion was an important goal of Session 1. At Session 2, group leaders should continue to establish group relationships. This short icebreaker is utilized to further promote the group cohesion process.

- Ask each child what he or she liked best about the first group session. Each child should be encouraged to talk about at least one thing that they enjoyed during the first session. In order to assist the children in this task, the group leader may want to model appropriate responses by being the first person to respond to this question.
- Take a 5-minute break. Remember to explain to the children what will occur during the break and what is expected of them during this time. Remind children that they must continue to follow all group rules during the break. Tell the children that they will be asked to sit down quietly and listen to the group leader explain the next activity following the break.

Goal 4: Help Children to Improve Homework Routines and to Identify Potential Reinforcers

- Introduce the *Fabulous Four Game*. This game provides an opportunity for children to describe their homework routines, including where, when, and with whom they complete their homework. Additionally, this game stimulates the children to brainstorm rewards that they would like to receive for appropriate homework behavior and performance. The purpose of the game is to prepare children to collaborate with their parents to develop a homework routine.

1. Divide the children into two teams.
2. Explain that the objective of the Fabulous Four Game is for the teams to provide four appropriate answers to each question asked.
3. Tell children that the teams will take turns being the first to answer questions.
4. Inform children that they will have 2 minutes to answer each question. During this time the team can write down their top four choices for answers. (Some children may require assistance with the actual writing.)
5. Explain that each team receives 1 point for each question they answer appropriately.
6. Use a colorful visual aid, such as a chart with drawings, to record points earned.

- Include the following questions in the Fabulous Four Game (sample game cards are provided in Appendix E):

1. Name four good places to do your homework.
2. Name four bad places to do your homework.

3. Name four materials that you need to have with you when you do your homework.
4. Name four good times to do your homework.
5. Name four things that you do when you are tired or frustrated from doing your homework.
6. Name four rewards you would like to receive when you complete your homework.

Goal 5: Discuss Group Homework Assignments

• Let the children know that their parents have been asked to sit down with them to discuss the ground rules for homework. Tell them that their parents will post these ground rules so that they are easily located. Stress that this activity can be very helpful in getting more work done in less time, so that the children and parents can move on to other daily activities.

• Inform the children that their parents will design a list of rewards for homework performance.

Conclusion of Session 2

• Tell each child the total number of points that he or she earned throughout the session. Instruct him or her to choose a prize (small, medium, or large) based on the number of total points earned.

• Emphasize positive behaviors displayed by each child in the session. Do not focus excessively on disruptive behaviors but simply exhort the children to keep up the good effort throughout the week and into the next session.

• End the group by reviewing the session's activities. For instance, review the importance of establishing a good homework routine.

SESSION 3: PROVIDING POSITIVE REINFORCEMENT

GOALS

1. Review group homework assignments.
2. Review token reinforcement system and establish personal goals.
3. Discuss the advantages of a token reinforcement system.
4. Discuss ways to identify reinforcers and promote productive behaviors.
5. Discuss group homework assignments.

This session is designed to help children better understand the use of positive reinforcement systems. In addition, the session should help children to verbalize what types of reinforcers would help motivate them to complete homework appropriately. Clinicians should prepare for this session by having the following materials available:

- *Supplies.* Two poster-sized pieces of paper for rules and agenda, name tags, prizes, snacks.
- *An integrity checklist for Session 3.* Clinicians should check each item on the checklist after it has been completed.

Goal 1: Review Group Homework Assignments

- Review the previous session's assignments with the parents and children during the initial 15 minutes of the session.
- Facilitate a discussion about the ground rules for homework that each family should have developed and posted since the last session.
- Provide praise for parents and children for their efforts to work collaboratively to design the homework ritual.

Goal 2: Review Token Reinforcement System and Establish Personal Goals

- Lead children into the child therapy room to begin the session.
- Review the rules and the token reinforcement system.
- Remind children that the reinforcement system is to begin at this point.
- Provide an overview of the session's activities.
- Help each child to set a personal goal for his or her behavior during the group. Each child's personal goal should address a specific behavior that the group leader and child agree should be a target for change. Examples of personal goals include: keeping one's hands to oneself, taking turns, participating in the group more frequently, and speaking louder so the entire group can hear.
- Evaluate the child's compliance with group rules, as well as the child's progress in meeting his or her personal goal, at each 15-minute checkpoint.

Goal 3: Discuss the Advantages of a Token Reinforcement System

- Ask children to identify how a token reinforcement system helps them to remain more focused and in better behavioral control during the group session.
- Ask what is the child's favorite thing about the token reinforcement system (i.e., they can earn a prize, they receive praise for positive behaviors, it reminds them to follow group rules, it makes the group more enjoyable).
- Ask children how the token reinforcement system could be improved.
- Take a 5-minute break. Remember to explain to the children what will occur during the break and what is expected of them during this time. Remind children that they must continue to follow all group rules during the break. Tell the children that they will be asked to sit down quietly and listen to the group leader explain the next activity following the break.

Goal 4: Discuss Ways to Identify Reinforcers and Promote Productive Behaviors

A role-play activity is introduced to provide an opportunity for children to identify and practice ways to negotiate with their parents and to identify various rewards for productive homework behavior. Children will be assigned to one of two teams and asked to create a short play of approximately 5 minutes in length.

- Divide the group into two teams.
- Briefly model a possible play that emphasizes reinforcers and productive behaviors.
- Find opportunities to praise children's efforts while they are enacting their plays.
- Refrain from offering corrective feedback as much as possible.
- Ask each team to perform one of the following plays for the other team:

    1. A play in which children discuss with their parents what rewards they would like to receive for completing their homework (i.e., praise, special privilege, a new toy).
    2. A play in which a child works very hard to pay attention to his or her homework and then receives verbal praise and a reward for being productive from his or her parents.

- After each team has acted out their play, have children reflect on the value of positive reinforcement systems (instead of punishment) in order to promote positive behaviors.

Goal 5: Discuss Group Homework Assignments

Let the children know that their parents will discuss with them, and then develop and implement, a token reinforcement system at home. Stress that the system is a terrific opportunity to make homework time better *and* for them to work toward rewards.

Conclusion of Session 3

- Tell each child the total number of points that he or she earned throughout the session. Instruct the child to choose a prize (small, medium, or large) based on the number of total points earned.
- Emphasize positive behaviors displayed by each child in the session. Do not focus excessively on disruptive behaviors but simply exhort the children to keep up the good effort throughout the week and into the next session.
- End the group by reviewing the session's activities. For instance, review the main points discussed about the positive features of token reinforcement systems.

SESSION 4: MANAGING TIME AND SETTING GOALS

GOALS

1. Review group homework assignments.
2. Review group rules and token reinforcement system.
3. Identify rewards for productive behaviors.
4. Help children understand the importance of time management and goal setting.
5. Introduce the Goal-Setting Tool to the children.
6. Discuss group homework assignments.

This session is designed to help children learn the benefits of time-management and goal-setting strategies for homework completion. Clinicians should prepare for this session by having the following materials available:

- *Supplies.* Two poster-sized pieces of paper for rules and agenda, name tags, prizes, "mystery" prize for the Fabulous Four Game, cards for the Fabulous Four Game, timer, snacks.
- *An integrity checklist for Session 4.* Clinicians should check each item on the checklist after it has been completed.

Goal 1: Review Group Homework Assignments

- Review the previous session's assignments with the parents and children during the initial 15 minutes of the session.
- Facilitate a discussion about the token reinforcement system that each family should have developed and enacted since the last session.
- Praise parents and children for their efforts to work collaboratively to design this reinforcement system.
- Request that the child complete the Children's Intervention Rating Profile (Appendix E).

Goal 2: Review Group Rules and Token Reinforcement System

- Lead children into the child therapy room to begin the session.
- Review the rules, token reinforcement system, and each child's personal goal.
- Remind children that the reinforcement system is to begin at this point.

Goal 3: Identify Rewards for Productive Behaviors

- Review the rules for the Fabulous Four Game (see Session 2 outline). Include the following questions in the Fabulous Four Game (sample cards are provided in Appendix E):

1. Name four rewards you have received for doing your homework.
2. Name four rewards you would like to receive for doing your homework.
3. Name four things that you do that will earn you rewards for homework.
4. Name four things that you do during homework that will not earn you rewards.

• Take a 5-minute break. Remember to explain to the children what will occur during the break and what is expected of them during this time. Remind children that they must continue to follow all group rules during the break. Tell the children that they will be asked to sit down quietly and listen to the group leader explain the next activity following the break.

Goal 4: Help Children Understand the Importance of Time Management and Goal Setting

• Present the children with the following problem in order to help them learn the concepts of time management and goal setting: "You have 100 math problems due in 4 days. As a group, I'd like you to plan how you will complete the problems."

• Facilitate a discussion of how the children will accomplish the task. Highlight the following time-management and goal-setting strategies:

1. Break the assignment down (i.e., complete only 25 problems per night).
2. Ask your parents for help if you do not understand portions of the assignment.
3. Give yourself a reward for each portion of the assignment that you finish correctly.

Goal 5: Introduce the Goal-Setting Tool to the Children

• Show children a copy of the Goal-Setting Tool (Appendix D) that their parents will be using with them over the next week.

• Emphasize that children first need to predict the number of problems that they think they can *complete* in each period of time and the number of problems they think they will answer *correctly* during this same period of time.

• Explain that children are to evaluate their product after working on each subunit. With assistance from their parents, they should fill in the amount of work *completed* and the amount of work performed *correctly* during each time period. Point out how children can use the Goal-Setting Tool to record information about their performance.

• Explain to children that they will earn points based on their ability to meet established goals. Demonstrate this by using the Goal-Setting Tool to predict percent completion and percent accuracy for an assignment of 25 math calculation problems.

Goal 6: Discuss Group Homework Assignment

• Let the children know that we have asked their parents to sit down with them to discuss setting time limits for completing their homework.

• Indicate that a Goal-Setting Tool will be used at home. Note that the technique will be a useful tool for breaking up homework and for earning rewards for complete and correct work.

Conclusion of Session 4

• Tell each child the total number of points that he or she earned throughout the session. Instruct the child to choose a prize (small, medium, or large) based on the number of total points earned.

• Emphasize positive behaviors displayed by each child in the session. Do not focus excessively on disruptive behaviors but simply exhort the children to keep up the good effort throughout the week and into the next session.

• End the group by reviewing the session's activities. For instance, review the main points discussed about the positive features of time management strategies and setting goals.

SESSION 5: USING PUNISHMENT SUCCESSFULLY

GOALS

1. Review group homework assignments.
2. Review group rules and token reinforcement system.
3. Discuss appropriate consequences for unproductive and disruptive behavior.
4. Discuss the upcoming conclusion of the group.
5. Discuss group homework assignment.

This session is designed to help children learn about consequences for unproductive and disruptive behavior. Clinicians should prepare for this session by having the following materials available:

• *Supplies.* Two poster-sized pieces of paper for rules and agenda, name tags, prizes, concentration cards (questions and picture cards), "mystery" prize for the winner of the concentration game, snacks.

• *An integrity checklist for Session 5.* Clinicians should check each item on the checklist after it has been completed.

Goal 1: Review Group Homework Assignments

- Review the previous session's assignments with the parents and children during the initial 15 minutes of the session.
- Facilitate a discussion about the Goal-Setting Tool that each family should have used since the last session.
- Ask both children and parents how well the Goal-Setting Tool worked and whether they enjoyed using this strategy.
- Ask the children what rewards they earned through use of the Goal-Setting Tool.

Goal 2: Review Group Rules and Token Reinforcement System

- Lead children into the child therapy room to begin the session.
- Review the rules, token reinforcement system, and each child's personal goal.
- Remind children that the token reinforcement system is to begin at this point.
- Provide an overview of the session's activities.
- Evaluate the child's compliance with group rules, as well as the child's progress in meeting his personal goal, at each 15-minute checkpoint.

Goal 3: Discuss Appropriate Consequences for Unproductive and Disruptive Behavior

- Review the instructions for the Homework Questions Concentration Game (see Session 1 outline). The questions for this version of the Homework Concentration Game should include the following (see Appendix E):

    1. What do your parents do when you pay attention and work hard while you are completing your homework?
    2. What do your parents do when you do not work hard during homework time?
    3. What do your parents do when you talk too much, argue, or get out of your chair during homework time?
    4. How would you feel about losing points for disruptive homework behavior?
    5. Are there some behaviors that you think your parents should punish?
    6. What are some fair ways for your parents to punish you?

- Take a 5-minute break. Remember to explain to the children what will occur during the break and what is expected of them during this time. Remind children that they must continue to follow all group rules during the break. Tell the children that they will be asked to sit down quietly and listen to the group leader explain the next activity following the break.

Goal 4: Discuss the Upcoming Conclusion of the Group

- Explain to the children that there are only two more sessions after this session, one the following week and the final session several weeks later.
- Process with the group any comments, questions, or concerns about the group's upcoming termination.

Goal 5: Discuss Group Homework Assignment

Let the children know that their parents have been asked to discuss with them how they will punish them for inappropriate behaviors (i.e., taking away points and privileges). Parents will identify specific behaviors that need to be changed and specific punishments that will occur if children break the rules at home.

Conclusion of Session 5

- Tell each child the total number of points that he or she earned throughout the session. Instruct the child to choose a prize (small, medium, or large) based on the number of total points earned.
- Emphasize positive behaviors displayed by each child in the session. Do not focus excessively on disruptive behaviors but simply exhort the children to keep up the good effort throughout the week and into the next session.
- End the group by reviewing the session's activities. For example, review the ideas generated in regard to parents removing points when a child misbehaves during homework time.

SESSION 6: INTEGRATING HOMEWORK SKILLS AND ANTICIPATING FUTURE PROBLEMS

GOALS

1. Review group homework assignments.
2. Review group rules and token reinforcement system.
3. Review the topics covered in the group.
4. Discuss how children feel about ending the group, and complete the farewell books.
5. Present each child with a certificate of achievement.
6. Discuss between-session assignment.

This session is designed to help children remember all of the techniques and strategies covered throughout the course of the group. In addition, this session helps children recognize their accomplishments through participation in Homework Success and allows them to learn appropriate ways of saying good-bye to friends. Clinicians should prepare for this session by having the following materials available:

- *Supplies.* Two poster-sized pieces of paper for rules and agenda, a small booklet with blank pages to serve as a "farewell book," prizes, snacks.
- *An integrity checklist for Session 6.* Clinicians should check each item on the checklist after it has been completed.

Goal 1: Review Group Homework Assignments

- Review the previous session's assignments with the parents and children during the initial 15 minutes of the session.
- Ask children and parents to describe the conversation they had to identify target behaviors for change and specific punishments for not following specified rules.
- Ask the children what rewards they earned through use of the Goal-Setting Tool.
- Request that the child complete the Children's Intervention Rating Profile (Appendix E).

Goal 2: Review Group Rules and Token Reinforcement System

- Lead children into the child therapy room to begin the session.
- Review the rules, token reinforcement system, and each child's personal goal.
- Remind children that the token reinforcement system is to begin at this point.
- Provide an overview of the session's activities.
- Evaluate the child's compliance with group rules, as well as the child's progress in meeting his or her personal goal, at each 15-minute checkpoint.

Goal 3: Review the Topics Covered in the Group

- Review the main topics covered in the group.
- To maximize the children's participation in this discussion, ask the children what they have learned in the group.
- When necessary, prompt the children by asking specific questions about what they have learned from the various group activities (e.g., role-play exercises, the Fabulous Four Game, and the Homework Concentration Game). This discussion should include a review of homework ground rules, positive reinforcement, time management and goal setting, and punishment.
- Provide examples to the children of how what they have learned will help them to make homework time more manageable and improve their relationships with their parents.
- Take a 5-minute break. Remember to explain to the children what will occur during the break and what is expected of them during this time. Remind children that they must continue to follow all group rules during the break. Tell the children that they will be asked to sit down quietly and listen to the group leader explain the next activity following the break.

Goal 4: Discuss How Children Feel about Ending the Group, and Complete the Farewell Books

- Explain to the children that they will be participating in an activity that is designed to help them finish the group.
- First, ask the children if they would like to express their feelings about the group coming to an end.
- Next, pass out a farewell book to each participant. Instruct participants to put their names on the front of their books and to spend a few minutes decorating the covers. Following this, ask each child to pass his or her book to the person on his or her left. Encourage each participant to write a note, draw a picture, or just sign his or her name in the other children's books. The books continue to be passed around until each participant has had the opportunity to sign all other participants' books.
- Remind children that there are two rules for this activity: (1) Everyone has to write or draw something (even if it's just a signature) in each book. (2) No negative messages or pictures are allowed in these books!
- Pay close attention to the time to ensure that everyone has the time to write in each of the books.

Goal 5: Present Each Child with a Certificate of Achievement

- Present each child with a certificate of achievement for successfully completing the Homework Success Program.
- As you hand each child his or her certificate, emphasize the positive gains made by the child through participation in the program.

Goal 6: Discuss Between-Session Assignment

- Let the children know that we have asked their parents to sit down with them to discuss the progress that they have made in completing their homework.
- Inform the children that the group will meet for a final session in several weeks.

Conclusion of Session 6

- Tell each child the total number of points that he or she earned throughout the session. Instruct the child to choose a prize (small, medium, or large) based on the number of total points earned.
- Emphasize positive behaviors displayed by each child in the session. Do not focus excessively on disruptive behaviors but simply exhort the children to keep up the good effort throughout the coming week and into the next session.
- End the group by reviewing the session's activities. For instance, mention the main components of the Homework Success Program and the importance of children continuing to work hard on the strategies they have learned through the program.

SESSION 7: PROVIDING FOLLOW-UP SUPPORT

GOALS

1. Review group homework assignment.
2. Review group rules and token reinforcement system.
3. Review the topics covered in the group.
4. Identify and role play how homework ground rules and token reinforcement systems are implemented.
5. Identify positive gains made by participants and anticipate future homework-related difficulties.

This follow-up session is designed to remind children of the techniques and strategies covered throughout the course of the group. In addition, this session helps children to recognize the accomplishments they have made through participation in Homework Success and to anticipate future homework-related difficulties. Clinicians should prepare for this session by having the following materials available:

- *Supplies.* Two poster-sized pieces of paper for rules and agenda, prizes, snacks.
- *An integrity checklist for Session 7.* Clinicians should check each item on the checklist after it has been completed.

Goals 1–3

- Because Goals 1–3 are identical to Goals 1–3 in Session 6, the reader is referred to the previous session.
- Take a 5-minute break. Remember to explain to the children what will occur during the break and what is expected of them during this time. Remind children that they must continue to follow all group rules during the break. Tell the children that they will be asked to sit down quietly and listen to the group leader explain the next activity following the break.

Goal 4: Identify and Role Play How Homework Ground Rules and Token Reinforcement Systems Are Implemented

- Review the instructions for conducting role plays (see Session 3 outline). Ask each team to design a play based on the following scenarios:

    1. Tommy is a 7-year-old boy who is in second grade. Tommy is having a very hard time completing his homework. Please help Tommy by making a list of homework ground rules for him to follow. Be sure to include rules for *where* and *when* Tommy should do his homework and *what materials* he needs to have with him when he does his homework.

2. Sally's parents are trying to set up a *token reinforcement system* to help motivate Sally to complete her homework without complaining. Identify what rewards she can earn for following homework ground rules and not complaining when completing her homework assignments.

Goal 5: Identify Positive Gains Made by Participants and Anticipate Future Homework-Related Difficulties

• Ask the children to identify two ways in which they have improved in doing their homework and relating to their parents since the start of the program.

• Ask each child to think about the types of homework difficulties that they may have in the future, along with strategies that may help them correct the problems.

• Take an active role in this discussion, in order to keep children engaged, positive, and future oriented.

Conclusion of Session 7

• Tell each child the total number of points that he or she earned throughout the session. Instruct the child to choose a prize based on the number of total points earned.

• Emphasize positive behaviors displayed by each child in the session. Do not focus excessively on disruptive behaviors but simply exhort the children to keep up the good work.

• End the group by mentioning the successes that each child has experienced over the course of the group, and wish each child good luck in the future.

ADDRESSING COMMON OBSTACLES

Many challenges can arise during group intervention programs, particularly when parent and child groups are conducted simultaneously. We describe below the most common obstacles (and recommended strategies to address each) that are likely to occur during the implementation of the child component of Homework Success. These issues can be broadly categorized as (1) problems with child behaviors, (2) variability in group composition, and (3) logistical challenges.

Problems with Child Behaviors

There are three common child behavioral difficulties that may be encountered when including children in Homework Success. Groups often contain one or more children who initially present as quiet and withdrawn. These children may be uncomfortable participating actively in the group and at times may even demonstrate a passive non-compliance, if their involvement is not proactively encouraged and supported. Also, there are often children who exhibit mild oppositionality or who may complain about their role in various group activities. Given the high comorbidity between ADHD and oppositional defiant disorder (ODD), this is a relatively common problem. Further, on occasion the group may include a child who is extremely oppositional or noncompliant. If the oppositional behavior is not managed well, it can greatly affect participants' enjoyment of the group.

In addressing behavioral issues in the group, it is important to pay attention to appropriate behaviors and selectively ignore the disruptive or attention-seeking behaviors exhibited by the noncompliant or nonparticipating child. A related approach is to encourage adaptive behaviors by providing high rates of positive feedback to other children in the group who are engaging in the appropriate behaviors. The noncompliant child who is seeking attention will often improve his or her behavior in order to receive the positive feedback given to the other children in the group. Another strategy that can be helpful is to make several attempts to engage the complaining or nonparticipating child in the session. These attempts can include making frequent eye contact, calling the child's name for a response even when his or her hand is not raised, pairing the child with a more cooperative group member during activities, and providing opportunities for the child to assume special roles. Approximations to adaptive behaviors should be reinforced.

The group leader can also utilize the child's personal goal to shape his or her behavior. In Session 3, each child identifies a personal goal to work on while participating in the sessions. The group leader should guide the child to select a goal that will be helpful to the child and the group. It is important that these goals be defined in a clear and concrete manner, even if they are approximations to ideal behaviors. For example, a goal for the noncompliant child might be to remain in his or her seat during the role play. A goal for the passive child might be to raise his or her hand at least one time during the group to provide a comment or ask a question.

If significant behavior problems occur among most of the children in the group, increasing the frequency with which points are given (i.e., shortening the time intervals) can be helpful. When addressing more severe oppositional behaviors exhibited within the group, it may be necessary to combine the positive reinforcement strategies described previously with restrictive strategies. For instance, a brief time-out can be an effective technique for children who continue to exhibit behavior that is disruptive to the group. On occasion, you may need to have a joint discussion with the child and his or her parents if noncompliant behaviors do not quickly improve.

Variability in Group Composition

Most groups will be highly diverse in composition. A group may include individuals who reflect a broad range of chronological ages, cognitive abilities, academic skill levels, and comorbid internalizing and externalizing difficulties. Such diversity can be a source of strength to the group, though several aspects need to be considered to maximize the usefulness of diversity within the child group.

Several strategies can be helpful in addressing issues of variability and diversity in group composition. First, it is recommended that group leaders match children within the group by pairing children of similar age and cognitive ability during structured activities. While matching children with similar characteristics, also attempt to pair children in a way that will enable them to complement each other's unique strengths. Second, create personal goals that will facilitate communication among diverse group members. Thus, if one child is substantially older than his or her groupmates but has difficulty expressing feelings, consider developing a personal goal that will enable the child to express his or her opinions. Third, assign special roles for children with differing strengths or weaknesses. Group leaders need to find a unique role for each child. Thus, a developmentally advanced child may be a "coleader" one week, and a cognitively limited or chronologically younger child may assist in holding up the poster of the group rules. Another individual may be an assistant when distributing snacks.

Logistical Challenges

Perhaps the most critical issue in conducting the child component of Homework Success is coordination with the adult group. Common obstacles in coordinating the child and parent groups include poor communication between adult- and child-group leaders, failure to complete weekly assignments, missed sessions, and parent- or child-training groups not ending on time.

There are a number of strategies that can address these challenges. Plan for regular and consistent communication between parent- and child-group leaders. Between sessions, group facilitators should meet together for a brief period to (1) outline the content of the first 15 minutes of the following session, (2) clearly define each facilitator's role in the combined group, as well as with individual families, (3) discuss the progress of each family, and (4) discuss the progress of each group to confirm that both child and parent groups are meeting weekly goals. Also, it is very useful to designate a case manager for each participating family prior to the start of Homework Success. Case managers discuss with parents issues pertaining to their progress, needs, and ability to follow through on program expectations. The case manager can also provide assistance with home–school communication.

Several other basic strategies can also facilitate better communication and planning between the group leaders. For instance, the leader of the parent group should inform the child-group leader if the parents have not adequately completed between-session assignments. This will help the child-group leader modify his or her teaching instructions when certain concepts are reviewed with the child. In addition, it is important that group leaders synchronize their watches and make every effort possible to end each session at the same time. Problems can arise if the parent group exceeds time limits and the child-group leader has to continue supervising children with ADHD-related behaviors who are ready to go home. Adherence to specified beginning and ending times also models structure and organization for participants.

MAKING THE PROGRAM MORE COMMUNITY RESPONSIVE

As noted earlier, Homework Success is ideally suited for use in school settings. Schools can offer a valuable resource in community partners, that is, residents of the surrounding community who can often be enlisted to assist with the implementation of the program. Enlisting community partners to serve as assistants in the child group can have many advantages. First, involving community members in this way is consistent with the movement toward establishing community-responsive, full-service schools (Dryfoos, 1994). Actively recruiting community partners sends a message to the community that the school wishes to involve community members in important school programs. Second, including community partners in providing intervention services will enable the program to be more meaningful and community responsive (Dowrick et al., in press; Manz et al., 2000). For instance, the inclusion of community partners often helps school personnel better understand community needs, improves communication between school personnel and community members pertaining to the nature of intervention services, and fosters more community support for school-based prevention and intervention services, particularly in low-income areas (Pumariega, 1996; Black & Krishnakumar, 1998). Third, engaging community partners as group assistants will foster the dissemination of the main principles and strategies of the program to members of the community. Fourth, community partners often have valuable talents and skills in working with families that will enhance the effectiveness of the Homework Success Program.

As group assistants, community partners contribute to the child group by aiding group leaders with any of the following: (1) establishing and implementing ground rules, (2) facilitating delivery of the session curriculum, (3) providing feedback to group leaders regarding problems that arise during the course of the program, and (4) assisting with detailed tasks that arise during each session (e.g., snacks, completing progress measures). Community partners may be recruited for participation in any number of ways. It is recommended that group leaders contact the school's parent–teacher association and/or advisory council to enlist community members. In addition, institutions such as churches and parent advocacy organizations may be useful resources. If appropriate, community partners may be given the option of serving as parent models in training videotapes and/or participating in in-session demonstrations of program principles and strategies.

CONCLUSIONS

Our experiences suggest that the success of the child component of Homework Success depends largely on the group leader's ability to conduct the child group in a systematic and thorough manner that is well coordinated with the parent-training group. There are a number of advantages to including the child component. First, conducting a child-training group allows children's homework and social difficulties to become normalized. Many children who have participated in the Homework Success Program have noted that they were relieved to know that other children also experience trouble with homework and/or with making and keeping friends. Second, as child participants learn homework strategies and begin to experience more homework-related successes, they tend to exhibit a greater sense of ownership and responsibility for their homework and behavioral difficulties. Third, the child-group experience can help children work more collaboratively with parents at home and allow them to see more clearly their parent's investment in their difficulties. As a result, parent–child conflicts may be reduced (see Habboushe et al., in press). Fourth, conducting the child group can also affect parents' perceptions of their children and influence their own follow-through with the recommended interventions. Finally, when parents see that their child is making the effort to examine his or her homework attitude and behaviors, parents are more willing to make the investment in learning alternative ways of helping their child.

## CHAPTER 15

Assessing Outcomes: Case Illustrations

SHEEBA DANIEL-CROTTY, DINA F. HABBOUSHE, JAMES L. KARUSTIS, AND THOMAS J. POWER

This chapter describes the outcomes of two groups of children who participated in Homework Success. These cases are presented to illustrate the range of outcomes that may occur in implementing this intervention program. A rigorous evaluation of Homework Success using carefully designed experimental group methods and single-subject designs is needed to validate the program. Our group is currently conducting a pretest–posttest control-group study with random assignment to groups that will provide a systematic evaluation of program effectiveness.

Each of the groups described in this chapter was composed of families coping with children who had been diagnosed with ADHD at an outpatient clinic in a tertiary-care pediatric hospital in a large metropolitan area. The diagnosis of ADHD was made on the basis of a structured diagnostic interview administered to the parents (Diagnostic Interview for Children and Adolescents; Reich, Leacock, & Shanfeld, 1995), as well as parent and teacher ratings of inattention and hyperactivity–impulsivity using the ADHD Rating Scale–IV (DuPaul, Power, et al., 1998). Each family was coping with a child who had significant problems with homework, as indicated by scores on the Homework Problem Checklist (HPC) that were greater than one standard deviation above the mean for children in elementary school (Anesko et al., 1987). The program was based in a clinic setting and included both a parent and child group. Parent groups were conducted by a licensed psychologist or predoctoral psychology intern; child groups were conducted by doctoral students. The procedures used in conducting the groups were very similar to those described in this manual.

After the families were enrolled in the program, and a week prior to Session 1, parents were sent a packet of questionnaires consisting of the HPC, the daily logs of homework performance, the Conflict Behavior Questionnaire (CBQ)—Parent Form, and the Parenting Stress Index (PSI)—Short Form. If two parents lived at home, the parent who reported spending the most time with the child during homework was asked to complete the questionnaires. In addition, the Academic Productivity subscale of the Academic Performance Rating Scale (APRS; DuPaul, Rapport, & Perriello, 1991) was sent to the teacher to complete prior to the first session. During Session 1, these questionnaires were collected from each family. Questionnaires (HPC, CBQ, PSI, APRS) were completed again in Session 6. During each session, the homework logs completed by parents during the previous week were collected.

To assess treatment acceptability, the Treatment Evaluation Inventory (TEI; Kelley et al., 1989)—Short Form was completed by the parents in Session 3 and again in Session 6. During each session, the group leader followed an integrity checklist that indicated the important components of content and process of the intervention. These checklists were very similar to the ones provided in Appendix B. In addition, each session was videotaped in order to monitor treatment integrity.

FINDINGS FOR GROUP 1

Group 1 consisted of five families. Four of the children were diagnosed with ADHD, combined type, and one child was diagnosed with ADHD, inattentive type. Based on the structured diagnostic interview administered to the parents, it was determined that three of the children who were diagnosed with ADHD, combined type, had a comorbid mood disorder, and two of those three also had a diagnosis of oppositional defiant disorder (ODD). The fourth child with ADHD, combined type, as well as the child who had ADHD, inattentive type, demonstrated no other comorbid diagnoses. All of the children demonstrated substantial homework difficulties. The children in this group were enrolled in grades 2 through 6 and had a mean age of 10 years. The intellectual functioning of participating children ranged from IQs of 91 to 126, with a mean IQ of 110, as assessed by the Wechsler Intelligence Scale for Children—Third Edition (WISC-III; Wechsler, 1991). Prior to and throughout the program one of the children was taking psychostimulant medication, and two of them were taking an antidepressant in addition to a stimulant. Four families were Caucasian and one family was African American. All families were of middle- to upper-middle socioeconomic status (SES), as determined by the Four-Factor Index of Social Status (Hollingshead, 1975).

Each of the families in Group 1 attended all seven sessions of the program. Videotapes of sessions were checked frequently to monitor intervention integrity. The group leaders consistently demonstrated adherence to over 95% of the tasks assigned to them for each group. No systematic problem with program implementation was noted.

The mothers completed outcome measures in four of the cases, and the father provided data for the fifth child. The group demonstrated marked reductions in homework problems from pretreatment to posttreatment. Scores on the HPC range from 0 to 60 with a mean of 10.5 and a standard deviation of 8.0 (Anesko et al., 1987). Prior to treatment, the mean score on the HPC for the group was 31.2; at posttreatment, the group mean decreased to 15.6, reflecting a reduction in parent-reported homework difficulties of approximately 2 standard deviations. The improvement in homework completion rates, as assessed by the parent-reported daily logs, was relatively small (an increase from 94% to 99%), primarily due to the fact that pretreatment levels of completion were generally very high. However, the mean percentage of homework accuracy increased from a rate of 72% at pretreatment to 83% at posttreatment. The group demonstrated essentially no change on the Academic Productivity subscale of the APRS, using normative data reported in Barkley (1991).

With regard to family functioning, there was a moderate reduction in parent–child conflict, as reported by parents on the CBQ. The difference from pretreatment to posttreatment was over one-half of a standard deviation, reflecting a moderate effect size (see Robin & Foster, 1989). There was essentially no change in reports of family stress as measured by the PSI. The acceptability of Homework Success was high at both midtreatment and posttreatment. On the TEI–Short Form yielding scores that range from 0 to 45, with high scores indicating greater acceptability, the group mean was 34.6 at midtreatment and 33.4 at posttreatment, reflecting positive perceptions about the reasonableness of the interventions throughout the program.

Table 15.1 displays scores on each outcome measure for the families that participated in Group 1. One of the cases is described in more detail below.

TABLE 15.1. Scores on Outcome Measures for Each of the Families in Group 1

Child	HPC	% complete	% accurate	APRS	CBQ	PSI
Child 1						
Pre	38	100	86	58	8	60
Post	8	100	97	51	2	50
Child 2						
Pre	27	81	86	39	5	34
Post	19	100	72	49	1	36
Child 3						
Pre	19	94	38	–	9	56
Post	15	94	85	–	11	62
Child 4						
Pre	35	100	79	44	9	50
Post	18	100	87	50	10	55
Child 5						
Pre	37	–	–	59	14	50
Post	18	–	–	50	13	57

Note. HPC (Homework Problem Checklist) scores are presented in raw-score format. Raw scores on the HPC range from 0 to 60, with a mean of 10.5 and a standard deviation of 8.0 (Anesko et al., 1987). Rates of work completion and accuracy were based on the daily logs of homework performance recorded by parents. APRS (Academic Productivity subscale of the Academic Performance Rating Scale; for normative data, see Barkley, 1991) scores are presented in T-score format. CBQ (Conflict Behavior Questionnaire–Parent Form) scores are presented in raw-score format. Raw scores on the CBQ range from 0 to 20, with a mean of 2.4 and a standard deviation of 2.8 (Robin & Foster, 1989). PSI (Total Stress score on the Parenting Stress Index–Short Form; Abidin, 1995) scores are presented in T-score format.

Case of Elizabeth

Elizabeth, a third-grade student, attended all seven sessions with both of her parents. Elizabeth was diagnosed with ADHD, combined type, ODD, and a mood disorder. She was taking a stimulant and antidepressant medication prior to, as well as throughout, the program. Elizabeth was a child who had difficulty completing work at home and at school, frequently made careless mistakes, often needed reminders to begin her work, and whined and complained often about homework. Although Elizabeth was of above-average intelligence (IQ = 115) and presented as a very verbal and motivated child, her teacher reported at the beginning of the program that she was only completing about 75% of her classwork at an accuracy rate of 75%. Prior to the start of Homework Success, Elizabeth's mother reported that they argued at least three times a week and that Elizabeth often did not listen to her mother. Elizabeth and her parents actively participated in the sessions. By their comments during the group, as well as their responses to between-session assignments completed, it was clear that the parents generally implemented the strategies that were presented in Homework Success. It is also important to note that Elizabeth's mother was experiencing some psychological distress and taking antidepressant medication.

At pretreatment, Elizabeth (Child 1 in Table 15.1) demonstrated significant homework difficulties, as reflected in a total score of 38 on the HPC, which is more than 3.5 standard deviations above the mean for elementary students. At posttreatment, she displayed a normalization of homework problems, that is, her score on the HPC was less than 1 standard deviation above the mean. Rate of homework completion was 100% at both pretreatment and posttreatment, but rate of work accuracy improved from 86% to 97%. Elizabeth demonstrated a slight reduction in scores on the Academic Productivity subscale of the APRS.

Elizabeth's mother reported a high level of negative communication and parent–child conflict on the CBQ at pretreatment, as indicated by a score that was greater than 2 standard deviations above the mean for nondistressed families. At posttreatment, however, Elizabeth's mother reported essentially no parent–child conflict. Stress related to parenting also decreased over the course of the program, from a T-score of 60 at pretreatment to a T-score of 50 at posttreatment.

FINDINGS FOR GROUP 2

All four children in Group 2 were diagnosed with ADHD; two had ADHD, combined type, and the other two had ADHD, inattentive type. In addition, each of the children had marked homework problems. None of the four children was diagnosed with a comorbid psychological disorder. The children were enrolled in grades 2 through 6, with a mean age of 10 years. Level of intellectual functioning ranged from 91 to 133, with a mean of 119, as assessed by the WISC-III. Two of the four children were taking psychostimulant medication prior to and throughout the program. Three families were Caucasian and one family was African American. All families were of middle-class to upper-middle-class SES, as determined by the Hollingshead scale.

Prior to treatment, the mean score on the HPC for the group was 27, which is about 2 standard deviations above the mean for children of this age. At posttreatment, the group mean on the HPC decreased to 13.0, which is less than 1 standard deviation above the mean. The improvement in homework completion rates was relatively small, primarily due to the fact that pretreatment levels of completion were generally high. The mean percentage of homework accuracy increased from a pretreatment level of 91% to a posttreatment level of 97%. There was no change in academic performance as reported on the APRS from pretreatment to posttreatment.

Parent reports of parent–child conflict on the CBQ decreased from 6.3 to 3.5, a full standard deviation. There was no change in family stress as reported on the PSI from pretreatment to posttreatment. Table 15.2 provides outcome data for each family in Group 2. One of these cases is discussed in some detail below.

Case of Alex

Alex, a fifth-grade student, attended all seven sessions with his mother. Alex was diagnosed with ADHD, combined type, and was taking stimulant medication prior to and throughout the program. Alex's homework-related problems consisted of failing to write down and bring home assignments, complaining that his homework was boring, and working in a disorganized fashion. Alex's mother reported that he often did not comply with requests and argued with her at least three times a week. Alex scored in the very superior range of intelligence, and his teacher reported that prior to the start of the program he completed 85% of his classwork at a 90% accuracy rate.

TABLE 15.2. Scores on Outcome Measures for Each of the Families in Group 2

Child	HPC	% complete	% accurate	APRS	CBQ	PSI
Child 6						
Pre	28	100	—	64	7	53
Post	7	100	100	62	5	52
Child 7						
Pre	26	100	94	47	4	38
Post	10	100	90	53	0	39
Child 8						
Pre	13	—	—	41	8	48
Post	10	—	—	34	5	46
Child 9						
Pre	42	100	88	47	6	61
Post	25	93	100	47	4	63

Note. HPC (Homework Problem Checklist) scores are presented in raw-score format. Raw scores on the HPC range from 0 to 60, with a mean of 10.5 and a standard deviation of 8.0 (Anesko et al., 1987). Rates of work completion and accuracy were based on the daily logs of homework performance recorded by parents. APRS (Academic Productivity subscale of the Academic Performance Rating Scale; for normative data, see Barkley, 1991) scores are presented in T-score format. CBQ (Conflict Behavior Questionnaire—Parent Form) scores are presented in raw-score format. Raw scores on the CBQ range from 0 to 20, with a mean of 2.4 and a standard deviation of 2.8 (Robin & Foster, 1989). PSI (Total Stress score on the Parenting Stress Index—Short Form; Abidin, 1995) scores are presented in T-score format.

At pretreatment, Alex (Child 6 in Table 15.2) demonstrated a score on the HPC that was 2 standard deviations above the mean for his agemates. At posttreatment he displayed a normalization of homework-related problems, that is, he scored less than 1 standard deviation above the mean on the HPC. His rate of completion of homework was 100% at both pretreatment and posttreatment. Unfortunately, data regarding homework accuracy were not available at baseline, but rate of accuracy at posttreatment was 100%. Functioning on the APRS was essentially unchanged throughout the program.

His mother's ratings of parent–child conflict decreased by about two-thirds of a standard deviation from pretreatment to posttreatment. Parenting stress was essentially unchanged.

CHAPTER 16

Conclusions

Homework performance has a significant impact on the academic functioning of children and adolescents. Homework has direct as well as indirect effects on academic achievement by shaping children's work habits and promoting parental involvement in school. Children with ADHD and related concerns, in particular, are highly vulnerable to problems with homework, which in turn can have a deleterious effect on their academic performance.

Homework also can have a strong impact on family functioning. Children with homework difficulties are often noncompliant and argumentative with parents when working on assignments. Some children spend an extraordinary amount of time doing homework, which can be a source of stress to parents and which may limit the amount of time parents have for other family matters, including time for play with the child, as well as time for their other children. Given that many children with ADHD are defiant and have problems with emotional regulation, the impact of homework-related problems on a family coping with ADHD can be especially disruptive.

Homework, therefore, is an important target of intervention for many children and families coping with problems related to ADHD. Improving homework performance has the potential to improve academic functioning, home–school communication, parent–child relationships, and family functioning.

Given the important roles of teachers, parents, and children in homework, programs to address homework problems should involve each of these parties fully in the process of intervention. The CBC model provides a very helpful framework for designing effective homework interventions. This model highlights the importance of actively engaging teachers, parents, and children in a collaborative problem-solving process to plan, implement, and evaluate a program of intervention. By applying principles of behavioral consultation and therapy, teachers, parents, and children are guided to address complex problems that affect both the school and family.

Effective interventions for homework problems must address both the antecedents and consequences of homework. Children with ADHD generally respond favorably to behavioral interventions. However, research has demonstrated that these children often require immediate, salient, concrete reinforcers, a high degree of variety in reinforcement, and response-cost procedures in order to improve their performance. Token reinforcement systems are particularly suited to this group of children because these interventions provide a mechanism for administering and removing salient, positive reinforcers with a high level of immediacy.

Homework Success applies a CBC model in engaging teachers, parents, and children in the process of designing, implementing, and evaluating behavioral interventions to address homework-related problems. Intervention is initiated by convening parents and teachers to identify homework difficulties, plan interventions, and discuss strategies for evaluating outcome. Throughout the course of intervention, parents receive guidance in how to collaborate effectively with teachers, and clinicians provide direct consultation to school professionals.

The primary method of delivering the Homework Success interventions is through group parent training. Research has affirmed repeatedly the effectiveness of group parent training in behavioral interventions. Advantages of group interventions are that they provide support to parents from their peers and opportunities for parents to assist each other in problem solving. Also, group interventions are often more cost effective than therapy provided to one family at a time.

Homework Success is also designed to include the child actively in the intervention process. We recommend that clinicians conduct a child group concurrent with the parent group. By so doing, clinicians can introduce strategies to children, facilitate their understanding and cooperation, and prepare them to work with their parents on these techniques at home.

This program can be provided in clinic, school, or community settings. Although each context has its advantages, we recommend the school or community center as a setting for intervention. Schools are accessible to families, afford many opportunities for home–school collaboration, and provide easy access to naturalistic data that are useful in monitoring progress. Community centers are often even more accessible and comfortable venues of service than are schools, particularly for families from urban settings.

A hallmark of effective intervention is the application of the procedures as intended. We strongly recommend that clinicians monitor carefully the integrity with which interventions are being applied by group leaders and the degree of parental adherence to between-session assignments. Integrity checklists for both the parent and child groups have been included in this manual to assist with the assessment of integrity.

Evaluation of program outcomes requires the use of a multimethod, multi-informant battery of measures to monitor progress and determine summative outcomes. Targets for assessment should include homework performance, academic functioning, and family functioning. We have recommended a variety of methods of assessing outcomes, including parent, teacher, and child ratings; examination of homework and classwork assignments; and review of existing, teacher-designed records.

In this manual we have presented detailed descriptions of the curriculum for each parent- and child-group session. Also, we have presented very specific homework assignments for parents to complete after each session. This information is presented to assist group leaders with the implementation of the program and to ensure that the intervention package is delivered with integrity. Although clinicians are encouraged to follow curriculum guidelines closely, it is critical that they deliver the service in a way that is comfortable for them and enables them to exercise their wonderful clinical talents.

At this point we have conducted the program with numerous groups of families. Rigorously controlled group and single-subject studies are still needed to evaluate the effectiveness of this program. Outcomes for the parents and children who have participated in Homework Success thus far have varied greatly from family to family and from one domain of assessment to another. For some families, this program has been sufficient to address their child's homework problems and related academic and family issues. However, for other families, this program was not sufficient, and referral for more intensive child and family therapy, often in combination with pharmacotherapy, was required. Given that so many families of children with ADHD-related problems have chronic concerns about homework, we recommend that clinicians assess outcomes over extended periods of time and be prepared to intervene when needed. By so doing, clinicians can provide a safety net for families who are particularly vulnerable to the challenges of homework.

APPENDIX A

Recruiting Handout and Letters

THE HOMEWORK SUCCESS PROGRAM

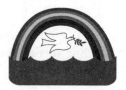

If you and your child are consistently having problems getting homework completed, or if your child's ability to stay focused is getting in the way of his or her homework productivity, the *Homework Success Program* may be just what is needed!

What is it? *Homework Success* is a group program designed to assist families who are experiencing significant problems related to homework and academic performance. We believe that *all* families have strengths that can be used to overcome such problems.

Who can participate? *Homework Success* is designed for families with children in grades 1 through 6. Children in this program have problems paying attention and controlling their behavior. Homework difficulties are extremely common among such children. We will provide a brief screening to determine if Homework Success is an appropriate program for your family's needs at this time. If this program is not well suited to your family's needs, we will provide guidance and resources to assist you in the right direction.

Will it take forever? Not at all! *Homework Success* is a seven-session group program, in which parents and children learn proven techniques for improving homework performance and for reducing parent–child conflict. It is a program intended to help good parents make homework time better.

Is a group the right place for this sort of thing? Most parents tell us that participating in Homework Success has helped them realize that they are not alone in their struggles. Many parents also report that participation in the program has helped them to see more clearly how strong their parenting skills are in some areas and how they can improve in areas that have been problematic for themselves and their children.

What is the cost? One of the benefits of a group program such as Homework Success is that it is much less expensive than individual therapy for homework problems. We will work closely with you regarding a reasonable payment plan.

We look forward to assisting you and your family!

SAMPLE RECRUITMENT LETTER FOR PHYSICIANS AND MENTAL HEALTH PROFESSIONALS

[**Logo and letterhead**]

THE HOMEWORK SUCCESS PROGRAM

Sylvia Collaborator, MD
1000 Referral Way
Springfield, ST 55555

[Date]

Greetings, Dr. Collaborator!

We wanted to let you know about a program that is to take place in our [clinic/school], beginning [date]. The **Homework Success Program** is designed to assist elementary school children (grades 1 through 6) and their parents or primary caregivers in improving homework and academic productivity and in improving parent–child relationships. Homework Success provides education regarding ADHD and behavioral management techniques such as positive reinforcement. Assistance is also provided regarding home–school communication.

Homework Success includes seven group sessions and is open to families of children with significant homework difficulties who are displaying impairing symptoms pertaining to inattention and/or hyperactivity–impulsivity. *Please note that an ADHD diagnosis is not mandatory for inclusion in the group.* Homework Success is founded on the belief that home–school collaboration is essential for school success. The group leader will be sure to remain in contact with you regarding issues pertaining to participants' [medication regimens and/or behavioral and academic progress]. We will provide a brief screening to determine families' appropriateness for participation. For those we determine to be in need of other services, we will provide information regarding intervention referrals and other resources.

We very much welcome the opportunity to collaborate with you in your patients' interests. *Accordingly, we are requesting that you inform families whom you feel may benefit from Homework Success about this program.* An information flyer has also been enclosed that can be given to parents and posted in your waiting room.

Please feel free to call us anytime regarding the program and potential participants. We can be reached here at [telephone and fax numbers, e-mail address].

Thank you in advance for your collaboration!

     Sincerely,

     [Clinician's name and title]

SAMPLE BRIEFING AND INTRODUCTORY LETTER FOR PUPIL SERVICES COORDINATORS

[Logo and letterhead]

THE HOMEWORK SUCCESS PROGRAM

Jesse Support, EdD
Director of Pupil Services
Springfield Public School District
2000 Referral Way
Springfield, ST 55555

[Date]

Dear Dr. Support:

We are pleased to announce the beginning of a brief group intervention program that may be of benefit to the families of many of the students in your district. The **Homework Success Program** is designed to assist elementary school children (grades 1 through 6) and their parents or primary caregivers in improving homework and academic productivity, and in improving parent–child relationships. Homework Success provides education regarding ADHD and behavioral management techniques such as positive reinforcement. Assistance is also provided regarding home–school communication.

Homework Success includes seven group sessions and is open to families of children with significant homework difficulties who are displaying impairing symptoms pertaining to inattention and/or hyperactivity–impulsivity. *Please note that an ADHD diagnosis is not mandatory for inclusion in the group.* Homework Success is founded on the belief that home–school collaboration is essential for school success. We will provide a brief screening to determine families' appropriateness for participation. For those we determine to be in need of other services, we will provide information regarding intervention referrals and other resources.

We very much welcome the opportunity to collaborate with you in your students' interests. We will be contacting you shortly to discuss any interest you feel there may be regarding our program. If it is so desired, we may also discuss the possibility of offering Homework Success in one of your schools. *If you feel the program may be appropriate and beneficial to the district's students, we would ask your written consent to distribute informative flyers and recruitment letters to school principals, counselors, and school psychologists.* An information flyer has also been enclosed for your consideration.

Please feel free to call us anytime with questions or other feedback regarding Homework Success. We can be reached here at [telephone and fax numbers, e-mail address]. Thank you in advance for your consideration!

Sincerely,

[Clinician's name and title]

SAMPLE BRIEFING AND INTRODUCTORY LETTER
FOR COUNSELORS, SCHOOL PSYCHOLOGISTS,
AND CHILD STUDY TEAM COORDINATORS

[Logo and letterhead]

THE HOMEWORK SUCCESS PROGRAM

Sheela Gupta, PhD
School Psychologist
South Springfield Elementary School
3000 Referral Way
Springfield, ST 55555

[Date]

Dear Dr. Gupta:

We have received a positive response from the school district's Pupil Services Director regarding a brief group intervention program that we are planning to conduct soon at our clinic. It is our belief that The **Homework Success Program** may be of significant benefit to many of your students and their parents.

Homework Success is designed to assist elementary school children (grades 1 through 6) and their parents or primary caregivers in improving homework and academic productivity and in improving parent–child relationships. Homework Success provides education regarding ADHD and behavioral management techniques such as positive reinforcement. Assistance is also provided regarding home–school communication.

Homework Success includes seven group sessions and is open to families of children with significant homework difficulties who are displaying impairing symptoms pertaining to inattention and/or hyperactivity–impulsivity. *Please note that an ADHD diagnosis is not mandatory for inclusion in the group.* The program is founded on the belief that home–school collaboration is essential for school success. We will provide a brief screening to determine families' appropriateness for participation. For those we determine to be in need of other services, we will provide information regarding intervention referrals and other resources.

We very much welcome the opportunity to collaborate with you in your students' interests. Please distribute the enclosed teacher packets, which include (1) a flyer describing the program; (2) a letter directed to the teachers requesting their suggestions about families who may be appropriate for the program; and (3) letters to be sent to the parents of identified students. Of course, we would also be glad to discuss families whom you feel would be appropriate for the program. Please feel free to call us anytime with questions or other feedback regarding Homework Success. We can be reached here at [telephone and fax numbers, e-mail address].

Sincerely,

[Clinician's name and title]

SAMPLE RECRUITMENT LETTER FOR PARENTS AND PRIMARY CAREGIVERS

[**Logo and letterhead**]

THE HOMEWORK SUCCESS PROGRAM

Dear Parents and Caregivers:

This letter is to inform you about a new group program that is to take place in our clinic for families of students in grades 1 through 6. You [and your child, if child group is to occur] are welcome and invited to participate. The program is called the **Homework Success Program**, and it is intended to assist you and your family to improve homework performance. We will offer strategies to get more work done in less time, education regarding attention problems, and guidelines on how to make homework time a positive experience for both you and your child. We will also assist you with any issues that may exist regarding home–school communication.

The **Homework Success Program** consists of seven group sessions. It is founded on the belief that collaboration between parents and schools is an essential part of a child's school success. We will be available to you for follow-up assistance as needed. We encourage you to read the enclosed flyer regarding the program and to contact us if you feel that your family may benefit from Homework Success. Most families have reported to us that they found Homework Success to be both enjoyable and productive.

The program will be starting on [date]. If you are interested in participating, or simply have some questions you would like to discuss, please contact us at [contact information]. If it appears that Homework Success is not the right program for your family at this time, we would be glad to provide information and support that may be of assistance.

       Sincerely,

       [Clinician's name and title]

Screening Instruments and Outcome Measures

ACADEMIC PERFORMANCE QUESTIONNAIRE

Instructions to teachers: The information provided on this form will assist in assessing this student's learning skills in relation to his or her classroom peers. Please answer the questions listed below. Thank you for your time and cooperation.

Student's name _____ School _____
Grade _____ Teacher's name _____
Type of class _____ Date completed _____

READING

Compared with the average students in your class, how well is this child able to **read orally**?
__ Well above average   __ Somewhat below average
__ At or just above average   __ Well below average

Compared with the average students in your class, how well is this child able to **comprehend what he or she reads**?
__ Well above average   __ Somewhat below average
__ At or just above average   __ Well below average

What are this student's specific problems, if any, in reading? _____
_____

Does this child participate in remedial reading? Yes __ No __
If yes, since when? ____ How often and for how long? ____
Type of remediation: __ Special education out-of-class support
                                  __ Special education in-class support
                                  __ Basic skills instruction
                                  __ Other school-based tutoring

MATHEMATICS

Compared with the average students in your class, how well is this student able to **perform math calculations**?
__ Well above average   __ Somewhat below average
__ At or just above average   __ Well below average

(cont.)

Compared with the average students in your class, how well is this student able to **perform math word problems**?

___ Well above average   ___ Somewhat below average
___ At or just above average   ___ Well below average

What are this student's specific problems, if any, in math? _____
_____
_____

Please estimate the percentage of written math work *completed* (regardless of accuracy) relative to classmates (circle one)   0–59%   60–69%   70–79%   80–89%   90–100%

Please estimate the *accuracy* of completed written math work (circle one)   0–59%   60–69%   70–79%   80–89%   90–100%

Does this child participate in remedial math?   Yes ___   No ___
If yes, since when? _____ How often and for how long? _____
Type of remediation: ___ Special education out-of class support
                              ___ Special education in class support
                              ___ Basic skills instruction
                              ___ Other school-based tutoring

WRITING

Compared with the average students in your class, how well is this child able to **write short stories or essays**?

___ Well above average   ___ Somewhat below average
___ At or just above average   ___ Well below average

What are this student's specific problems, if any, in writing? _____
_____
_____

Please estimate the percentage of written language arts work *completed* (regardless of accuracy) relative to classmates (circle one)   0–59%   60–69%   70–79%   80–89%   90–100%

Please estimate the *accuracy* of completed written language arts work (circle one)   0–59%   60–69%   70–79%   80–89%   90–100%

HOMEWORK

What are this student's specific problems, if any, regarding homework? _____
_____
_____

Please estimate the percentage of homework *completed* (circle one)   0–59%   60–69%   70–79%   80–89%   90–100%

How would you rate the quality of this student's homework?   A   B   C   D   E   F

OTHER COMMENTS _____
_____
_____

HOMEWORK PERFORMANCE QUESTIONNAIRE

Student's name _____ Date of birth __/__/__ Grade __
Gender (circle) Male Female Completed by _____
Your relationship to student _____ Date completed __/__/__

Please check only one for each statement	0	1	2	3
Please rate the child's behavior for each item below.	Never	At times	Often	Very often
1. Leaves necessary homework materials at school				
2. Does not know what the assignments are				
3. Lies about having completed homework at school				
4. Does homework in a distracting location				
5. Needs many reminders to begin homework				
6. Needs constant supervision to remain on task				
7. Argues or complains				
8. Becomes frustrated easily				
9. Rushes through assignments, making careless errors				
10. Fails to submit work to teacher				
11. Difficulties with homework causes problems in my relationship with this child				
12. Difficulties with homework with this child cause problems in my relationship with other family members				

(cont.)

Average daily *time* (in minutes) spent on homework *over the past* 2 *weeks* (circle)

Mathematics	None	1–10	11–20	21–40	41–60	61–90	91–120	more than 2 hrs
Reading assignments	None	1–10	11–20	21–40	41–60	61–90	91–120	more than 2 hrs
Language/spelling	None	1–10	11–20	21–40	41–60	61–90	91–120	more than 2 hrs
Other	None	1–10	11–20	21–40	41–60	61–90	91–120	more than 2 hrs

Percentage of work *completed* for each subject *over the past* 2 *weeks* (circle)

Mathematics	0–25%	26–50%	51–70%	71–80%	81–90%	91–100%
Reading assignments	0–25%	26–50%	51–70%	71–80%	81–90%	91–100%
Language/spelling	0–25%	26–50%	51–70%	71–80%	81–90%	91–100%
Other	0–25%	26–50%	51–70%	71–80%	81–90%	91–100%

Quality of your child's homework *over the past* 2 *weeks* (circle)

Math accuracy	A	B	C	D	E	F
Reading comprehension	A	B	C	D	E	F
Writing neatness	A	B	C	D	E	F
Writing content	A	B	C	D	E	F
Spelling	A	B	C	D	E	F

ATTENTION-DEFICIT/HYPERACTIVITY DISORDER KNOWLEDGE AND OPINION SURVEY (AKOS)

Child's name _____ Your name _____ Date _____

The purpose of this survey is to help us better understand your knowledge of and opinions about attention-deficit/hyperactivity disorder (ADHD). The first part consists of a series of true–false statements. Circle T if you believe the statement is true or right. Circle F if you think the statement is false or wrong.

PART 1

1. Most children with ADHD have problems with attention when they become teenagers. T F
2. Children with ADHD can be OK in some situations (such as at home) and can be distractible and disruptive in others (such as at school). T F
3. Special diets, like the Feingold diet, have been scientifically proven to improve the symptoms of most people with ADHD. T F
4. Tests given in a psychologist's office are necessary for making the diagnosis of ADHD. T F
5. Medication often reduces a child's tendency to be aggressive with others at school. T F
6. ADHD may sometimes be inherited (passed along in the family). T F
7. Children with ADHD almost always meet national and state standards for learning disabilities. T F
8. Boys and girls have similar rates of ADHD. T F
9. Children with ADHD are usually brighter than those without ADHD. T F
10. In most cases, medication will help a child achieve better grades in school. T F
11. There is a medical test that is very effective in identifying children with ADHD. T F
12. For most children with ADHD, psychological treatments are not as effective as medication in improving attention and reducing disruptive behaviors. T F
13. The medication(s) used to treat ADHD are of little benefit when children reach adolescence or adulthood. T F
14. There is reliable evidence that ADHD is often caused by having too much sugar in a child's diet. T F
15. Children who are hyperactive at the age of 3 almost always become identified as having ADHD by the age of 7. T F
16. There are new medications available that are more effective and safer than previous medications such as Ritalin. T F
17. The diagnosis of ADHD can be made if symptoms first develop at the age of 10. T F

(cont.)

PART 2

For each of the following statements, please relate your own opinions by circling the number that appears most like *your* views. Assume that your child *does* have ADHD, even if this has not yet been confirmed.

18. I believe that medication could help my child with ADHD

1	2	3	4	5	6
Strongly Disagree	Disagree	Disagree Somewhat	Agree Somewhat	Agree	Strongly Agree

19. Our family could benefit from counseling sessions to learn how to cope better with our child with ADHD.

1	2	3	4	5	6
Strongly Disagree	Disagree	Disagree Somewhat	Agree Somewhat	Agree	Strongly Agree

20. When my child misbehaves, other people usually tell me I do not know how to discipline him or her the correct way.

1	2	3	4	5	6
Strongly Disagree	Disagree	Disagree Somewhat	Agree Somewhat	Agree	Strongly Agree

21. I think that scheduling problems would make it difficult for us to arrange counseling appointments.

1	2	3	4	5	6
Strongly Disagree	Disagree	Disagree Somewhat	Agree Somewhat	Agree	Strongly Agree

22. Doctors should take into account parents' opinions about what is best for their child when making treatment recommendations.

1	2	3	4	5	6
Strongly Disagree	Disagree	Disagree Somewhat	Agree Somewhat	Agree	Strongly Agree

23. Health problems in the family will make it difficult for us to get involved with counseling at this time.

1	2	3	4	5	6
Strongly Disagree	Disagree	Disagree Somewhat	Agree Somewhat	Agree	Strongly Agree

24. I would be reluctant to start our child on a medication for ADHD.

1	2	3	4	5	6
Strongly Disagree	Disagree	Disagree Somewhat	Agree Somewhat	Agree	Strongly Agree

25. In general, I think I know how to handle my child pretty well.

1	2	3	4	5	6
Strongly Disagree	Disagree	Disagree Somewhat	Agree Somewhat	Agree	Strongly Agree

26. My child's behavior is so difficult to control that sometimes I feel like a failure as a parent.

1	2	3	4	5	6
Strongly Disagree	Disagree	Disagree Somewhat	Agree Somewhat	Agree	Strongly Agree

27. I believe that medication for ADHD is basically safe and has only minor side effects.

1	2	3	4	5	6
Strongly Disagree	Disagree	Disagree Somewhat	Agree Somewhat	Agree	Strongly Agree

28. I would be reluctant to have our family attend counseling sessions to find ways to better work with our child with ADHD.

1	2	3	4	5	6
Strongly Disagree	Disagree	Disagree Somewhat	Agree Somewhat	Agree	Strongly Agree

29. This is not a good time for our family to begin counseling.

1	2	3	4	5	6
Strongly Disagree	Disagree	Disagree Somewhat	Agree Somewhat	Agree	Strongly Agree

30. Other people are pretty impressed with the way I handle my child.

1	2	3	4	5	6
Strongly Disagree	Disagree	Disagree Somewhat	Agree Somewhat	Agree	Strongly Agree

31. A doctor's recommendations are generally based upon sound scientific evidence and should be followed regardless of my personal feelings or beliefs.

1	2	3	4	5	6
Strongly Disagree	Disagree	Disagree Somewhat	Agree Somewhat	Agree	Strongly Agree

32. I could use some professional counseling to help my family and me deal with my child with ADHD in better ways.

1	2	3	4	5	6
Strongly Disagree	Disagree	Disagree Somewhat	Agree Somewhat	Agree	Strongly Agree

33. Payment problems will make it difficult for our family to follow through with counseling, if recommended, at the present time.

1	2	3	4	5	6
Strongly Disagree	Disagree	Disagree Somewhat	Agree Somewhat	Agree	Strongly Agree

34. I am confident that a medication is safe for my child if a doctor who is knowledgeable about ADHD recommends it.

1	2	3	4	5	6
Strongly Disagree	Disagree	Disagree Somewhat	Agree Somewhat	Agree	Strongly Agree

(cont.)

35. I would not agree to the use of medication for my child even if dependable experts were recommending it.

1	2	3	4	5	6
Strongly Disagree	Disagree	Disagree Somewhat	Agree Somewhat	Agree	Strongly Agree

36. I believe that our family will have trouble finding the time to get involved in counseling at this time.

1	2	3	4	5	6
Strongly Disagree	Disagree	Disagree Somewhat	Agree Somewhat	Agree	Strongly Agree

37. Medical experts generally know the best treatments for ADHD.

1	2	3	4	5	6
Strongly Disagree	Disagree	Disagree Somewhat	Agree Somewhat	Agree	Strongly Agree

38. I have a good understanding of my child's emotional needs.

1	2	3	4	5	6
Strongly Disagree	Disagree	Disagree Somewhat	Agree Somewhat	Agree	Strongly Agree

39. Our family should have no difficulty traveling to and from counseling sessions.

1	2	3	4	5	6
Strongly Disagree	Disagree	Disagree Somewhat	Agree Somewhat	Agree	Strongly Agree

40. Family therapy would probably be helpful to us.

1	2	3	4	5	6
Strongly Disagree	Disagree	Disagree Somewhat	Agree Somewhat	Agree	Strongly Agree

41. Counseling would be too expensive for my family to get involved with at this time.

1	2	3	4	5	6
Strongly Disagree	Disagree	Disagree Somewhat	Agree Somewhat	Agree	Strongly Agree

42. Television and newspaper reports about Ritalin and ADHD have made me very uneasy and frightened about giving my child medication.

1	2	3	4	5	6
Strongly Disagree	Disagree	Disagree Somewhat	Agree	Agree	Strongly Agree

43. If a doctor recommends that we go for counseling as a family, I would go despite my (or my partner's) reluctance to do so.

1	2	3	4	5	6
Strongly Disagree	Disagree	Disagree Somewhat	Agree Somewhat	Agree	Strongly Agree

Thank you very much for your time and effort in filling out this questionnaire.

ATTENTION-DEFICIT/HYPERACTIVITY DISORDER KNOWLEDGE AND OPINION SURVEY (AKOS) SCORING SHEET

Child's name _____ Date _____
Relationship of rater to the child _____

PART 1: KNOWLEDGE SCALE
(circle correct answers)

1. T	7. F	13. F
2. T	8. F	14. F
3. F	9. F	15. F
4. F	10. F	16. F
5. T	11. F	17. F
6. T	12. T	

Total score: ____

Norms	M	SD
Mothers (n = 87)	11.0	2.4
Fathers (n = 63)	10.9	2.2

PART 2: OPINION FACTORS
(write in number circled; items marked with an asterisk should be scored in reverse: 6 = 1, 5 = 2, 4 = 3, 3 = 4, 2 = 5, 1 = 6).

Medication acceptability	Counseling acceptability	Counseling feasibility
18 ____	19 ____	21* ____
24* ____	26 ____	33* ____
27 ____	28* ____	39 ____
34 ____	29* ____	41* ____
35* ____	32 ____	
42* ____	36* ____	
	40 ____	
	43 ____	

Factor score: ____   ____   ____

NORMS

	M	SD		M	SD		M	SD
Mothers	25.0	6.2		37.1	7.1		14.9	4.4
Fathers	23.8	6.2		34.7	4.6		15.2	3.1

Note. The norms were generated from 87 mothers and 63 fathers of children referred to an ADHD evaluation and treatment program based in a university-affiliated children's hospital.

DAILY HOMEWORK LOG (FOR PARENTS)

Name of child: _____

Parent(s) completing log: _____

Week of: _____

Subject	Monday				Tuesday				Wednesday				Thursday				Fri/Sat/Sun			
	No. of prob-lems	No. com-pleted	No. correct	Time	No. of prob-lems	No. com-pleted	No. correct	Time	No. of prob-lems	No. com-pleted	No. correct	Time	No. of prob-lems	No. com-pleted	No. correct	Time	No. of prob-lems	No. com-pleted	No. correct	Time

ACADEMIC PERFORMANCE RATING SCALE

Student _____ Date _____

Age ___ Grade ___ Teacher _____

For each or the below items, please estimate the above student's performance over the *past week*. For each item, please circle *one* choice only.

1. Estimate the percentage of written math work *completed* (regardless or accuracy) relative to classmates.	0–49% 1	50–69% 2	70–79% 3	80–89% 4	90–100% 5
2. Estimate the percentage of written language arts work *completed* (regardless of accuracy) relative to classmates.	0–49% 1	50–69% 2	70–79% 3	80–89% 4	90–100% 5
3. Estimate the *accuracy* of completed written math work (i.e., percent correct of work done).	0–49% 1	50–69% 2	70–79% 3	80–89% 4	90–100% 5
4. Estimate the accuracy of completed written language arts work (i.e., percent correct of work done).	0–49% 1	50–69% 2	70–79% 3	80–89% 4	90–100% 5
5. How consistent has the quality of this child's academic work been over the past week?	Consistently poor 1	More poor than successful 2	Variable 3	More successful than poor 4	Consistently successful 5
6. How frequently does the student accurately follow teacher instructions and/or class discussion during *large-group* (e.g., whole class) instruction?	Never 1	Rarely 2	Sometimes 3	Often 4	Very often 5
7. How frequently does the student accurately follow teacher instructions and/or class discussion during *small-group* (e.g., reading group) instruction?	Never 1	Rarely 2	Sometimes 3	Often 4	Very often 5

(cont.)

8. How quickly does this child learn new material (i.e., pick up novel concepts)	Very slowly 1	Slowly 2	Average 3	Quickly 4	Very quickly 5
9. What is the quality or neatness of this child's handwriting	Poor 1	Fair 2	Average 3	Above average 4	Excellent 5
10. What is the quality of this child's reading skills?	Poor 1	Fair 2	Average 3	Above average 4	Excellent 5
11. What Is the quality of this child's speaking skills?	Poor 1	Fair 2	Average 3	Above average 4	Excellent 5
12. How often does the child complete written work in a hasty fashion?	Never 1	Rarely 2	Sometimes 3	Often 4	Very often 5
13. How frequently does the child take more time to complete work than his/her classmates?	Never 1	Rarely 2	Sometimes 3	Often 4	Very often 5
14. How often is the child able to pay attention without you prompting him/her?	Never 1	Rarely 2	Sometimes 3	Often 4	Very often 5
15. How frequently does this child require your assistance to accurately complete his/her academic work?	Never 1	Rarely 2	Sometimes 3	Often 4	Very often 5
16. How often does the child begin written work prior to understanding the directions?	Never 1	Rarely 2	Sometimes 3	Often 4	Very often 5
17. How frequently does this child have difficulty recalling material from a previous day's lessons?	Never 1	Rarely 2	Sometimes 3	Often 4	Very often 5
18. How often does the child appear to be staring excessively or "spaced out"?	Never 1	Rarely 2	Sometimes 3	Often 4	Very often 5
19. How often does the child appear withdrawn or tend to lack an emotional response in a social situation?	Never 1	Rarely 2	Sometimes 3	Often 4	Very often 5

SCORING INSTRUCTIONS FOR THE ACADEMIC PERFORMANCE RATING SCALE

The subscales of the Academic Performance Rating Scale (DuPaul et al., 1991) consist of the following items:

Academic Success: 3, 4, 5, 8, 10, 11, 17
Impulse Control: 9, 12, 16
Academic Productivity: 1, 2, 3, 4, 5, 6, 7, 13, 14, 15, 18, 19

To compute the subscale score, add the ratings given to each item on the subscale. Note that ratings for items 12, 13, 16, 17, 18, 19 must be reverse-scored so that high ratings correspond with positive academic functioning.

Means and Standard Deviations for the APRS by Grade and Gender

Grade	Total Score	Academic Success	Impulse Control	Academic Productivity
Grade 1 (n = 82)				
Girls (n = 40)	67.02 (16.27)	23.92 (7.37)	9.76 (2.49)	44.68 (10.91)
Boys (n = 42)	71.95 (16.09)	26.86 (6.18)	10.67 (2.82)	46.48 (11.24)
Grade 2 (n = 91)				
Girls (n = 46)	72.56 (12.33)	26.61 (5.55)	10.15 (2.70)	47.85 (7.82)
Boys (n = 45)	67.84 (14.86)	25.24 (6.15)	9.56 (2.72)	44.30 (10.76)
Grade 3 (n = 92)				
Girls (n = 43)	72.10 (14.43)	25.07 (6.07)	10.86 (2.65)	47.88 (9.35)
Boys (n = 49)	68.49 (16.96)	25.26 (6.53)	9.27 (2.67)	45.61 (11.89)
Grade 4 (n = 79)				
Girls (n = 38)	67.79 (18.69)	24.08 (7.56)	10.36 (2.91)	44.26 (11.96)
Boys (n = 41)	69.77 (15.83)	25.35 (6.50)	9.83 (2.77)	45.71 (10.22)
Grade 5 (n = 79)				
Girls (n = 44)	73.02 (14.10)	26.11 (6.01)	10.76 (2.34)	48.36 (9.05)
Boys (n = 35)	63.68 (18.04)	23.14 (7.31)	8.69 (2.82)	42.40 (12.47)
Grade 6 (n = 70)				
Girls (n = 31)	74.10 (14.45)	26.59 (6.26)	10.79 (2.25)	48.77 (9.13)
Boys (n = 39)	65.24 (12.39)	23.75 (5.90)	9.05 (2.35)	43.59 (8.19)

Note. Standard deviations are in parentheses. From DuPaul, Rapport, and Perriello (1991). Copyright 1991 by the National Association of School Psychologists. Reprinted by permission of the publisher.

CONFLICT BEHAVIOR QUESTIONNAIRE—PARENT VERSION

Name of parent: _____ Date: _____
I am completing this form regarding my child _____.

Think back over the last 2 weeks at home. The statements below have to do with you and your child. Read the statement and then decide if you believe that the statement is true. If it is true, then circle **True**, and if you believe the statement is not true, circle **False**. You must circle either True or False, but never both for the same item. Please answer all items. Answer for yourself, without talking it over with anyone.

True False   1. My child is easy to get along with.

True False   2. My child is well behaved in our discussions.

True False   3. My child is receptive to criticism.

True False   4. For the most part, my child likes to talk to me.

True False   5. We almost never seem to agree.

True False   6. My child usually listens to what I tell him/her.

True False   7. At least three times a week, we get angry with each other.

True False   8. My child says I have no consideration of his/her feelings.

True False   9. My child and I compromise during arguments.

True False   10. My child often doesn't do what I ask.

True False   11. The talks we have are frustrating.

True False   12. My child often seems angry at me.

True False   13. My child acts impatient when I talk.

True False   14. In general, I don't think we get along very well.

True False   15. My child almost never understands my side of an argument.

True False   16. My child and I have big arguments about little things.

True False   17. My child is defensive when I talk to him/her.

True False   18. My child thinks my opinions don't count.

True False   19. We argue a lot about rules.

True False   20. My child tells me he/she thinks I am unfair.

CONFLICT BEHAVIOR QUESTIONNAIRE—CHILD VERSION

Name of child: _____ Date: _____
I am completing this form regarding my parent _____.

Think back over the last 2 weeks at home. The statements below have to do with you and your parent who helps you most with homework. Read the statement and then decide if you believe that the statement is true. If it is true, then circle **True**, and if you believe the statement is not true, circle **False**. You must circle either True or False, but never both for the same item. Please answer all items.

True	False	1. My parent doesn't understand me.
True	False	2. My parent and I sometimes end our arguments calmly.
True	False	3. We almost never seem to agree.
True	False	4. I enjoy the talks we have.
True	False	5. When I state my opinion, my parent gets upset.
True	False	6. At least three times a week, we get angry with each other.
True	False	7. My parent listens when I need someone to talk to.
True	False	8. My parent is a good friend to me.
True	False	9. My parent says I have no consideration for him/her.
True	False	10. At least once a day we get angry with each other.
True	False	11. My parent is bossy when we talk.
True	False	12. My parent understands me.
True	False	13. The talks we have are frustrating.
True	False	14. My parent understands my point of view, even if he/she doesn't agree with me.
True	False	15. My parent seems to be always complaining about me.
True	False	16. In general, I don't think we get along very well.
True	False	17. My parent screams a lot.
True	False	18. My parent puts me down.
True	False	19. If I run into problems, my parent helps me out.
True	False	20. I enjoying spending time with this parent.

SCORING INSTRUCTIONS FOR THE CONFLICT BEHAVIOR QUESTIONNAIRE

Parent Version

Add 1 point for each of the following items answered True: 5, 7, 8, 10, 11, 12, 13, 14, 15, 16, 17, 18, 19, 20.

Add 1 point for each of the following items answered False: 1, 2, 3, 4, 6, 9.

Child Version

Add 1 point for each of the following items answered True: 1, 3, 5, 6, 9, 10, 11, 13, 15, 16, 17, 18.

Add 1 point for each of the following items answered False: 2, 4, 7, 8, 12, 14, 19, 20.

HOMEWORK SUCCESS EVALUATION INVENTORY

Name (optional): _____

Date: _____

Please indicate the extent of your agreement or disagreement with each of the following statements by circling the number that best describes your opinion. Refer to the following scale when making your judgments.

1	2	3	4	5	6
Strongly disagree	Disagree	Disagree a little	Agree a little	Agree	Strongly agree

1. The strategies of Homework Success make sense to me.

    1   2   3   4   5   6

2. I believe this program can be helpful to my child and family.

    1   2   3   4   5   6

3. The Homework Success strategies are reasonable and fair.

    1   2   3   4   5   6

4. The approaches used in this program can have positive effects and no real negative side effects on my child and family.

    1   2   3   4   5   6

5. I think that most families would find the Homework Success strategies to be practical and useful.

    1   2   3   4   5   6

6. This type of program can make a positive difference for families coping with homework problems.

    1   2   3   4   5   6

7. Making a commitment to this program is worth the time and effort.

    1   2   3   4   5   6

HOMEWORK SUCCESS PROGRAM EVALUATION SCALE

Name (optional): _____

Date: _____

SECTION A. Please rate how helpful each topic of the program has been for you and your family.

1. Understanding ADHD and how it has an effect on homework performance

1	2	3	4	5
Not helpful	A little helpful	Helpful	Very helpful	Extremely helpful

2. Establishing a consistent homework ritual (i.e., when, where, what)

1	2	3	4	5
Not helpful	A little helpful	Helpful	Very helpful	Extremely helpful

3. Giving effective instructions and commands

1	2	3	4	5
Not helpful	A little helpful	Helpful	Very helpful	Extremely helpful

4. Providing positive reinforcement

1	2	3	4	5
Not helpful	A little helpful	Helpful	Very helpful	Extremely helpful

5. Managing time and goal setting

1	2	3	4	5
Not helpful	A little helpful	Helpful	Very helpful	Extremely helpful

6. Using punishment successfully

1	2	3	4	5
Not helpful	A little helpful	Helpful	Very helpful	Extremely helpful

7. Integrating skills and anticipating future problems

1	2	3	4	5
Not helpful	A little helpful	Helpful	Very helpful	Extremely helpful

(cont.)

SECTION B. Please rate each aspect of the program regarding how helpful it has been for you and your child.

8. Organization of the group

1	2	3	4	5
Not helpful	A little helpful	Helpful	Very helpful	Extremely helpful

9. The parent–teacher meeting at the outset of the program

1	2	3	4	5
Not helpful	A little helpful	Helpful	Very helpful	Extremely helpful

10. The way that group leaders managed time during the sessions

1	2	3	4	5
Not helpful	A little helpful	Helpful	Very helpful	Extremely helpful

11. Group leader's knowledge of the program's topics

1	2	3	4	5
Not helpful	A little helpful	Helpful	Very helpful	Extremely helpful

12. Group leader's attention to my needs

1	2	3	4	5
Not helpful	A little helpful	Helpful	Very helpful	Extremely helpful

13. The handouts

1	2	3	4	5
Not helpful	A little helpful	Helpful	Very helpful	Extremely helpful

14. The parent homework assignments

1	2	3	4	5
Not helpful	A little helpful	Helpful	Very helpful	Extremely helpful

15. The opportunity to share experiences with and learn from other parents

1	2	3	4	5
Not helpful	A little helpful	Helpful	Very helpful	Extremely helpful

16. When appropriate, the group experience provided to my child

1	2	3	4	5
Not helpful	A little helpful	Helpful	Very helpful	Extremely helpful

SECTION C. Other Feedback.

17. What aspects of the program have been the most helpful to you?

18. What suggestions do you have for us that may be helpful for future groups?

Thank you very much for taking the time to provide us with this feedback. All the members of the Homework Success team wish you good luck in your future endeavors!

APPENDIX C

Integrity Checklists for Parent Group

SESSION 1: INTEGRITY CHECKLIST

Date: _____ Group leader: _____

CONTENT

❑ Have materials ready.
    ❑ Name tags and markers
    ❑ Handouts 1–5
    ❑ Daily Homework Logs
    ❑ Conflict Behavior Questionnaire

❑ Ask parents to complete and wear name tags.

❑ Group leader introduces self to participants.

❑ Ask parents to introduce themselves and give their reasons for participating.

❑ Generate discussion of homework problems each parent is experiencing.

❑ (If child group is being conducted) Encourage children to introduce themselves and to participate in discussion. Then have them leave room to go to their group.

❑ Describe the rationale for using baseline and progress measures; have parents complete CBQ.

❑ Discuss goals and format of program, including ground rules for group.

❑ Discuss parent–teacher consultation meeting.

❑ Distribute Handout 1; encourage discussion of program goals.

❑ Discuss Conjoint Behavioral Consultation model.

❑ Distribute Handout 2; highlight importance of completing between-session assignments.

❑ Promote hope by acknowledging frustration and by referring to program's past successes.

❑ Distribute Handout 3; discuss specifics of ADHD.

❑ Break

❑ Distribute Handout 4; discuss relation between ADHD and homework problems, including need to limit time spent on homework.

❑ Distribute Handout 5; emphasize importance of using assignment sheet.

❑ Distribute Daily Logs; discuss parent assignments to be completed prior to next session.

PROCESS

❑ Did each parent participate in the group discussions?

❑ Was the group leader responsive to each family's needs?

SESSION 2: INTEGRITY CHECKLIST

Date: _____ Group leader: _____

CONTENT

❑ Have materials ready.
  ❑ Name tags and markers
  ❑ Daily Homework Logs
  ❑ A-B-C Worksheets (Handout 6)
  ❑ Handouts 7–9
  ❑ Outcome measures (Homework Performance Questionnaire, Homework Success Evaluation Inventory)

❑ Collect Daily Homework Logs.

❑ Review between-session assignments from previous session.

❑ (If applicable) Include children in discussion of assignments; then have children leave room.

❑ Distribute Handout 6; generate discussion about antecedents and consequences of behavior.

❑ Ask a parent to volunteer to do a functional assessment of a homework problem behavior; write on board, using A-B-C system.

❑ Distribute Handout 7; describe basics of homework ritual.

❑ Distribute Handout 8; assess participant understanding of use of this worksheet; practice.

❑ Break

❑ Distribute Handout 9; review characteristics of effective instructions.

❑ Invite parents to discuss specifics of delivering instructions, including potential obstacles.

❑ Discuss between-session assignments; emphasize importance of use of Family Assignments sheet.

PROCESS

❑ Did each parent participate in group discussion?

❑ Did each parent discuss between-session assignments from the previous week?

❑ Was the group leader responsive to each family's needs this week?

BETWEEN SESSIONS 2 AND 3

❑ Contact teacher and make arrangements to collect outcome data; thank teacher for collaboration.

SESSION 3: INTEGRITY CHECKLIST

Date: _____ Group leader: _____

CONTENT

❑ Have materials ready.
   ❑ Name tags and markers
   ❑ Daily Homework Logs
   ❑ A-B-C Worksheets
   ❑ Handouts 10–12

❑ Review between-session assignments.

❑ (If applicable) Include children in discussion of assignments; then have children leave room.

❑ Review issues pertaining to parental noncompliance with assignments.

❑ Elicit examples from participants of their use of positive reinforcement; praise such usage.

❑ Distribute Handout 10; discuss principles of positive reinforcement.

❑ Emphasize importance of using positive reinforcement relative to punishment.

❑ Review potential obstacles to consistently using positive reinforcement.

❑ Discuss types of positive reinforcers.

❑ Assist parents in developing individualized positive reinforcement systems.

❑ Break

❑ Distribute Handout 11; describe rationale for using Homework Rewards Worksheet.

❑ Distribute Handout 12; present detailed discussion of token/point system principles and techniques.

❑ Introduce CISS-4 acronym; underscore importance of each CISS-4 component.

❑ Discuss between-session assignments.

❑ Remind parents to continue using A-B-C Worksheets and Daily Homework Logs.

❑ Remind parents to give points every 15 minutes.

❑ Remind parents to call between sessions if needed.

PROCESS

❑ Did each parent participate in group discussion?

❑ Did each parent discuss between-session assignments from the previous week?

❑ Was the group leader responsive to each family's needs this week?

SESSION 4: INTEGRITY CHECKLIST

Date: _____ Group leader: _____

CONTENT

❑ Have materials ready.

    ❑ Name tags and markers
    ❑ Daily Homework Logs, A-B-C Worksheets, and Handout 13
    ❑ Outcome measures: Homework Performance Questionnaire and Homework Success Evaluation Inventory

❑ Collect Daily Homework logs; distribute additional logs and A-B-C Worksheets.

❑ Review between-session assignments.

❑ (If applicable) Include children in discussion of assignments; then have children leave room.

❑ Have parents complete outcome measures.

❑ Discuss family experiences implementing token/point systems; troubleshoot problems with each parent using an A-B-C Worksheet.

❑ Address problems pertaining to compliance with between-session assignments.

❑ Review importance of limiting time spent on homework; troubleshoot potential obstacles, including parental beliefs.

❑ Discuss benefits of setting realistic goals for homework time, completion, and accuracy.

❑ Break

❑ Distribute Handout 13; introduce and explain in detail each principle and intervention technique.

❑ Role play use of Goal-Setting Tool; model by working with a child, or use videotape, if possible.

❑ Have participants practice using GST, with children, if possible.

❑ Underscore importance of using GST and remaining persistent, emphasizing benefits of its use.

❑ Discuss between-session assignments.

PROCESS

❑ Did each parent participate in group discussion?

❑ Did each parent discuss between-session assignments from the previous week?

❑ Was the group leader responsive to each family's needs this week?

BETWEEN SESSIONS 4 AND 5

❑ Consult with teacher, including review of Homework Success principles and interventions, as well as discussion of child's homework progress; thank teacher for continued collaboration.

❑ Obtain outcome data from teacher.

SESSION 5: INTEGRITY CHECKLIST

Date: _____ Group leader: _____

CONTENT

❑ Have materials ready.

    ❑ Name tags and markers
    ❑ Daily Homework Logs and A-B-C Worksheets
    ❑ Handouts 14–15

❑ Collect Daily Homework logs; distribute additional logs and A-B-C Worksheets.

❑ Review between-session assignments, including discussion with teacher.

❑ (If applicable) Include children in discussion of assignments; then have children leave room.

❑ Discuss experiences using GST; troubleshoot problems with implementation.

❑ Distribute Handout 14; ensure that parents understand use of these worksheets.

❑ Break

❑ Distribute Handout 15; present rationale for using punishment successfully.

❑ Discuss basic principles and techniques for using punishment, referring to Handout 15.

❑ Describe potential adverse side effects of using punishment.

❑ Remind parents of CISS-4 principles; generate discussion of their experiences using the principles.

❑ Emphasize continued use of GST, Daily Homework Logs, A-B-C Worksheets.

❑ Discuss between-session assignments.

❑ Remind parents that the next session is the last one prior to the follow-up meeting; encourage participants to work on integrating skills they have developed over the course of the program.

PROCESS

❑ Did each parent participate in group discussion?

❑ Did each parent discuss between-session assignments from the previous week?

❑ Was the group leader responsive to each family's needs this week?

SESSION 6: INTEGRITY CHECKLIST

Date: _____ Group leader: _____

CONTENT

❑ Have materials ready.

    ❑ Name tags and markers
    ❑ Daily Homework Logs and A-B-C Worksheets
    ❑ Handout 16
    ❑ Outcome measures: Conflict Behavior Questionnaire, Homework Success Evaluation Inventory
    ❑ Materials for group celebration

❑ Collect Daily Homework logs and A-B-C Worksheets; distribute additional logs and A-B-C Worksheets.

❑ Review between-session assignments.

❑ Review use of daily assignment book.

❑ (If applicable) Include children in discussion of assignments; then have children leave room.

❑ Collect GSTs that have been completed; praise adherence and troubleshoot problems.

❑ Generate discussion regarding progress, continuing problems, and commentary regarding the program.

❑ Ask parents to complete the Homework Performance Questionnaire.

❑ Compare issues noted on this HPQ with baseline HPQ; discuss ways to modify procedures to address persisting problems.

❑ Distribute Handout 16; review each topic and request parent input pertaining to ways that they can modify strategies to suit their family's needs.

❑ Break

❑ Introduce formula for success concept; provide examples on board and assist parents with developing their own success formulas.

❑ Remind parents of importance of attending follow-up session.

❑ Ask parents to complete outcome measures.

❑ Conduct celebration, with child participants in room (if applicable); emphasize specific progress points.

PROCESS

❑ Did each parent participate in group discussion?

❑ Did each parent discuss between-session assignments from the previous week?

❑ Was the group leader responsive to each family's needs this week?

BETWEEN SESSIONS 6 AND 7

❑ Make arrangements with teachers to collect outcome data; inform teacher of status of program, and request an update regarding children's progress.

SESSION 7: INTEGRITY CHECKLIST

Date: _____ Group leader: _____

CONTENT

❑ Have materials ready.
  ❑ Name tags and markers
  ❑ Daily Homework Logs and A-B-C Worksheets
  ❑ Handout 17
  ❑ Outcome measures: Homework Performance Questionnaire, Conflict Behavior Questionnaire, Homework Success Evaluation Inventory
  ❑ Diplomas

❑ Collect Daily Homework logs and A-B-C Worksheets; distribute additional logs and A-B-C Worksheets.

❑ Review between-session assignments, include discussion of formula for success.

❑ Review use of daily assignment book.

❑ (If applicable) Include children in discussion of assignments; then have children leave room.

❑ Discuss GSTs that have been completed; praise adherence and troubleshoot problems.

❑ Review core components of Homework Success Program; provide reminders of basic principles.

❑ Identify progress made and assist parents with troubleshooting problems.

❑ Ask parents to select one homework problem; assist them with conducting a functional assessment using an A-B-C Worksheet; use board to facilitate this process.

❑ Distribute Handout 17; encourage them to use this handout and to join and participate in support and educational organizations such as CHADD.

❑ Discuss with group the possibility of convening follow-up booster session in 2–3 months, if desired.

❑ Inform parents that they may contact the group leader with questions or issues subsequent to the conclusion of the program.

❑ Ask parents to complete outcome measures.

❑ Ask parents to talk about one or two things in the program that they have found to be helpful.

❑ (If applicable) Have children reenter the room; issue diplomas to parents and (if applicable) children.

PROCESS

❑ Did each parent participate in group discussion?

❑ Did each parent discuss between-session assignments since Session 6?

❑ Was the group leader responsive to each family's needs this week?

AFTER SESSION 7

❑ Contact teachers to obtain follow-up data and comments regarding children's progress; thank teacher for collaboration.

APPENDIX D

Parent Handouts

WELCOME TO THE HOMEWORK SUCCESS PROGRAM!

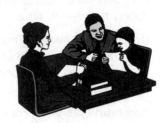

We welcome you and your child to the Homework Success Program. This program is designed to assist your family in coping with the challenges of homework, so that your child can succeed better academically and so that you can enjoy a more satisfying relationship with your child. Many families have reported that the strategies learned in this program have enabled them to change homework from a time of conflict and stress to an opportunity for collaboration and problem solving.

OUR APPROACH

We use what is called a *Conjoint Behavioral Consultation Model* in this program. By *Conjoint* we mean that all individuals who are important to the child play a role in intervention. Specifically, the individuals (and their roles) involved in this team are:

1. **Parents:** Learn and apply the program's behavioral strategies.
2. **Child:** Learn the strategies and cooperate with parents in applying them.
3. **Group leader:** Teach the behavioral strategies and provide consultation to team members.
4. **Teachers:** Provide frequent feedback to child and parents. Make accommodations based on collaborative problem solving with the parents and group leader.
5. **Physicians:** Prescribe and monitor medication as needed. Consult with team members as required.

It is important that within each of these roles we are all working together for the common goals of increasing homework productivity and decreasing your child's behavioral problems.

Behavioral refers to an approach that focuses on identifying and targeting environmental influences on a child's actions. Specifically, we are interested in examining and changing the events that occur before and after a problem behavior and that may serve to provoke or maintain a problem. The key to a behavioral approach is to focus on events that can be changed and not to focus on intrinsic personality issues that are very difficult to change.

Consultation refers to the process of promoting collaboration among team members to work adaptively and solve problems by effectively using behavioral strategies in different settings.

Please bring this folder to each session, as we will be distributing worksheets and educational handouts each week. For the first few weeks we request that you wear your name tag. In order to get the most out of the group, we also ask that you follow these guidelines:

1. **Please arrive at each session on time.** One of the basic principles of Homework Success is to begin homework at the same time each day. Therefore it is important that you *model timeliness* for your child by being ready to begin the group on time. We will be meeting on the same evening each week for 90

(cont.)

minutes. The group will meet for 6 consecutive weeks, with a booster session to follow 4 weeks later (a total of 7 sessions). In the booster session, the group meets to discuss successes and problems each participant has encountered using the tools provided in the Homework Success Program. Beverages and snacks will also be provided.

2. **Participate!** By expressing your concerns and voicing your opinions, you will gain much support from one another and will have a greater opportunity to learn and to address the needs of your family.

3. **Listen!** In this group you will discover that you are not alone. Parents repeatedly tell us how much they have benefited from listening to the experiences of others as to how they deal with the problems faced during homework time.

4. **Do your homework.** This is an active, goal-directed program. Parents who are committed to improving the quality of their child's homework consistently do their Homework Success assignments. One way to ensure that you do not become overly frustrated is to allow us to assist you in troubleshooting problems with assignments.

5. **Communicate with your child's teacher.** Frequent and collaborative home–school communication is essential to achieve the goals of this program. Ask questions of your child's teacher, and be sure to let him or her know how your child is progressing regarding the Homework Success goals.

6. **Call us.** Do not hesitate to call us if you experience problems when doing your between-session assignments during the week.

7. **Respect confidentiality.** A key requirement of Homework Success is that you not discuss other families' problems and issues outside of the session room.

8. **Hang in there.** Although many families begin to experience positive effects from the program right away, benefits will usually tend to become more evident as the group unfolds. So while you and your child work hard and try to remain patient, we urge you to hang in there.

9. **Be hopeful!** Addressing homework difficulties is a very challenging process. However, we are confident that if you consistently attend, listen, actively participate, and work very hard to apply these strategies, you will observe some very positive changes in your child's homework productivity, as well as in your relationship with your child.

10. **Try to enjoy the process!** Strange as this may sound while you and your child are experiencing homework problems and conflicts, the process of working on improving homework time does not have to be painful. We strongly encourage you to take note of the gains that you make and to celebrate them.

WEEKLY FAMILY ASSIGNMENTS

Week	Assignment	Day or days completed

ATTENTION-DEFICIT/HYPERACTIVITY DISORDER (ADHD):
BASIC FACTS

1. **Is there more than one type of ADHD?** The disorder now referred to as ADHD has undergone many changes over the years in terms of how it is classified. The primary categories of symptoms are *(a) inattention,* (b) *impulsivity,* and (c) *hyperactivity,* which are classified into three ADHD subtypes: predominantly inattentive type, predominantly hyperactive–impulsive type, and combined type (i.e., inattentive, hyperactive, impulsive). As you can see, it is not necessary for a child to display symptoms of hyperactivity or impulsivity in order to receive an ADHD diagnosis. In fact, approximately 30–40% of children receiving an ADHD diagnosis are in the predominantly inattentive subtype.

2. **If a person has the symptoms, does that mean he or she *has* ADHD?** The occurrence of ADHD symptoms in itself is not enough to receive an ADHD diagnosis. The following criteria must also be met:

   a. Symptoms must be present in more than one setting, such as *both* home and school.
   b. The child must have some sort of clinical impairment associated with the symptoms. In other words, *the symptoms must cause a significant problem* in the child's academic, social, and/or behavioral functioning.
   c. Some symptoms must have been present before age 7.

3. **Where does ADHD come from?** First, let's dispel some common rumors.

   a. ADHD is not caused by faulty parenting.
   b. ADHD is not caused by poor teachers.
   c. ADHD is not caused by the junk food that your child eats.

   - We are *not* claiming here that parenting and teaching practices cannot *affect* a child's functioning (more on this later). In fact, one of our guiding principles for treatment is that effective parenting and teaching practices can help increase appropriate behaviors, and decrease undesirable behaviors.
   - Although research has repeatedly failed to support a significant relationship between diet and ADHD, we recognize that diet can be a contributing factor to problems in some children with ADHD.
   - ADHD tends to be inherited.
   - There is increasing evidence that ADHD is usually a neurologically based disorder entailing deficits in self-regulation. Put simply, this means that those areas of the brain that play a significant role in concentrating, planning, and controlling impulses may be underactive.
   - ADHD is more common in boys than in girls (about a 3-to-1 ratio).
   - Despite all of the attention this disorder gets in the press about its overdiagnosis and epidemic proportions, the prevalence of ADHD has been found to be about 5% of school-aged children.

4. **Who is qualified to diagnose my child?** Professionals with expertise in development and behavioral principles are most qualified to assess whether or not a child has ADHD. Such persons may include psychologists, psychiatrists, neurologists, and pediatricians. In order to conduct a thorough assessment,

such professionals should compile information about a child's development and functioning across situations. Brief observations in a psychologist's or physician's office do not provide enough information to accurately assess ADHD.

5. **Could my child have a problem that looks like ADHD but is really something else?** There are two main points to take into account regarding this question.

    a. **ADHD imposters.** Symptoms of ADHD may appear in children who actually have other problems. Some common examples:
        *   A child who is depressed or anxious may have problems concentrating but may not have ADHD.
        *   A child whose learning problems have not been adequately addressed may very well have a difficult time sitting still and paying attention, mainly because he or she cannot understand what is being taught.
        *   Many children who do not follow directions or are disruptive in class may have oppositional defiant disorder (ODD) or another behavior disorder.
        *   Finally, stressful events in a child's life may take up so much energy that there is a decreased ability to concentrate or control oneself. For example, a child whose parent is seriously ill may be preoccupied about the parent and may consequently not be focusing in school.

    b. **Comorbidity.** This term is used when an individual has more than one diagnosable condition. There are many conditions that frequently exist along with ADHD. For instance:
        *   About 50% of children with ADHD also have ODD.
        *   Approximately 20% of those with ADHD have an anxiety or mood disorder.
        *   About 25% of children with ADHD have specific learning disabilities.

    In order to lessen the risk of misdiagnosing and therefore inappropriately treating a child, it is important to assess for learning, mood, and other behavioral problems, as well as environmental and family stressors.

6. **Will this go away?** Hyperactivity tends to decrease when children reach adolescence. However, many children continue to display symptoms of inattention and impulsivity into adulthood. Given proper treatment, the majority of children with ADHD can develop skills to cope with their symptoms and eventually become successful in important areas of their lives. It is critical that parents shift their perspective and approach from attempting to "cure" their children to focusing on "managing" the symptoms.

7. **What can be done?** An effective treatment plan generally includes behavioral and school interventions and, in many cases, the use of medication. In order to manage ADHD, it is necessary to identify and change practices in a child's environment that sustain problems. This usually requires parent education about the disorder, as well as training in behavioral strategies, such as giving effective commands and consequences. School personnel also need to use behavioral techniques in the classroom, such as daily home–school notes (with home-based rewards), changes in seating, increased structure, frequent positive feedback, and the use of peer tutors. Individual therapy with children is rarely sufficient by itself, although it may be included as needed in an overall family behavioral therapy program.

8. **What about medication?** At least 75% of children with an ADHD diagnosis display behavioral improvements from the use of psychostimulant medications such as Ritalin, Dexedrine, Adderall, or Cylert. Parents are advised to consult with their child's physician regarding possible benefits and negative side effects of psychostimulants. There are a number of misconceptions related to the use of medications for treating ADHD that need to be addressed. The realities are the following:

    a. Research shows that children who are prescribed psychostimulant medication for ADHD are no more likely than other teenagers to abuse substances in adolescence.
    b. A positive response to psychostimulant medication does not indicate that a child has ADHD. In fact

(cont.)

many individuals without ADHD demonstrate improvements in concentration, impulse control, and work completion while on the medication.

c. Children's needs change over the course of development. Although many children with ADHD continue to take medication into adolescence and adulthood, this is not inevitable. It should *not* be assumed that once prescribed medication, children will require it through adulthood. One of the positive things about most psychostimulants is that *trial periods* on and off medication can be used to determine if the medication is producing beneficial effects.

d. Ritalin and chemically similar medications are psychostimulants, not sedatives. Therefore, when appropriately prescribed and administered, most children should not appear sedated.

9. **How about biofeedback, herbal remedies, and diet?** Research has not offered adequate support for these interventions for ADHD, although research in the future will help to clarify whether they may be useful. A combination of behavioral, instructional, and medical interventions is usually considered the most effective approach in the treatment of ADHD. Currently, there is a lack of evidence regarding the effectiveness of these other approaches.

You can probably think of other questions having to do with ADHD. You and your child are encouraged to ask us and your physician. In addition, there are many other resources available to assist in building your knowledge base. Children and Adults with Attention Deficit Disorders (CHADD) is an educational/support organization for families of persons with ADHD (800-233-4050). At the close of the Homework Success Program we will provide you with a list of resources. Bookstores usually sell many books on ADHD. Current bestsellers include *Taking Charge of ADHD* by Russell Barkley, *Power Parenting for ADD/ADHD* by Grad Flick, and *ADHD/Hyperactivity* by Michael Gordon.

SOME WAYS ADHD IS RELATED TO HOMEWORK PROBLEMS

Examples of ADHD symptoms	Observed behaviors	Common resulting problems
Forgetfulness	Leaves homework book at school.	Homework does not get completed.
		Homework is done inaccurately or carelessly.
Restlessness	Does not stay seated during homework.	Daily arguments with parents.
		Failing grades at school.
Daydreaming	Does not remain focused during homework.	Homework takes too long.
		Parents become frustrated.
Avoiding tasks that require effort	Attempts to get out of doing work.	Child becomes discouraged.
		Teacher lowers expectations.
		Siblings and classmates are neglected.
Distractibility	Does not remain on task.	Child gets "bad kid" reputation.
Appearing not to be listening	Problems following instructions.	Child's positive behaviors are overlooked.
		Adults play "Blame Game."
		Siblings and classmates tease child.
Talking excessively	Disturbs others; fails to listen to adults during key instructional moments.	

HOMEWORK ASSIGNMENT SHEET

Assignments for the week of: _____			
Day:	**Subject**	**Assignment**	**Due**
			Complete ☐
			Complete ☐
			Complete ☐
			Complete ☐
			Complete ☐
			Complete ☐

Things to remember:

Teacher's signature: _____

HOMEWORK ASSIGNMENT SHEET (Sample)

Assignments for the week of: 11/29/99

Day:	Subject	Assignment	Due
Monday	Reading	Read Chapter 4, pages 5 to 10	Tuesday 11/25
		Answer Questions 1 to 5, page 11	Complete ☒
	Math	Do all problems on attached sheet	Tuesday 11/25
			Complete ☒
	Social Studies	No Homework Assignment	
			Complete ☐
	Science	Do Section II of Atoms Project	Wednesday 11/26
			Complete ☒
	Art	Cut out picture of space shuttle and bring in to class	Tuesday 11/25
			Complete ☒
			Complete ☐

Things to remember:

Teacher's signature: Mrs. Jill Johnson

HOMEWORK A-B-C WORKSHEET

	Antecedents	Behavior	Consequences	Outcome
	What happened immediately before?	What did your child do?	What did you do?	What was your child's response to the consequence?
Monday				
Tuesday				
Wednesday				
Thursday				
Friday/Weekend				

ESTABLISHING THE HOMEWORK RITUAL

1. **Location, location, location!** Location refers to the ***where*** of homework. Negotiate this with your child. There should be few distractions (e.g., television, siblings, toys). However, your child should be situated where you can provide the necessary supervision, such as being able to enforce time limits and provide spot checks. For instance, the bedroom may be relatively distraction free, but may not be close enough for you to provide necessary help.

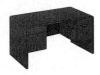

2. **I wanna watch TV for a while!** Structure is absolutely essential when working with a child with ADHD. Set up a homework schedule and stick to it. This is the first aspect of the ***when*** of homework. Try to begin work at the same time each day. There are many things to consider here. First, if your child takes a quick-acting medication (such as Ritalin) after school, you may wish to wait 30 minutes before beginning homework. Consider when your child is able to pay attention best after school, as this will vary from child to child. You will also have to take into account meals and after-school activities such as sports. Try to allow your child enough play time at the end of homework to serve as a reward for getting work done.

3. **Time limits are vital.** Establish reasonable time limits for homework and do not let homework exceed these limits. Using time limits may initially seem uncomfortable to many parents who are anxious about their child "falling behind." It has been our experience that many children initially seem to fall behind a little when time limits are instituted. But the payoff is usually superb! You will learn to set goals to reinforce your child for greater and greater levels of productivity. As you practice setting time limits, you will eventually become very comfortable with this strategy. Most children with ADHD who are held to time limits by their parents will become more productive, even though they are gradually spending less time on homework.

4. **"Gimme a break!"** This should be agreed upon ahead of time. Only a minute or two! We recommend a fun minute of jumping up and down. Alternately, the break time can be used to go to the bathroom or to get a drink of water.

5. **Use a timer.** This should be set for the amount of time until the break. For some children you may have to keep the timer out of view to minimize distraction.

6. **Use a homework kit.** Be sure to have a homework kit in good shape prior to beginning work. This should include the following, if they are appropriate to your child's needs and developmental level (you and your child may wish to include additional items):

Pencils	Pencil sharpener	Pens (if appropriate)
Paper	Scissors	Eraser
Calculator	Timer (see above)	Adhesive tape

Praise your child if she or he has the homework kit already prepared. You may wish to make a game of initially obtaining the materials and assembling the homework kit. A number of parent/teacher educational stores sell colorful containers specifically designed to hold homework materials.

(cont.)

---

7. **The teacher told me we don't have any homework tonight!** How can you be sure you know what homework your child needs to complete? This is part of the ***what*** of homework. Most students are sup-posed to use some form of a Homework Assignment Sheet. Make this part of the homework ritual. For instance, one rule may be that your child shows you the Homework Assignment Sheet as soon as he or she walks through the door and greets you. This should be signed by the teacher, with "No Assignment" written in and signed when appropriate. If this is completed, give the first re-ward! If not, have a backup plan ready. Many schools have homework hotlines. Your child should also have the telephone numbers for at least three class-mates. The *what* of homework also refers to bringing home the books that are needed to complete as-signments. There may be a space on the Homework Assignment Sheet to indicate that your child has the proper materials for homework.

Those are the basics of the Homework Ritual. A few other things to remember:

8. **Remember to keep your roles clear.** Your child will at times need your help with understanding the homework material. This is part of your role of homework tutor. Keep this job distinguished from your role as homework supervisor. Provide assistance to your child before and after an assignment. Your pri-mary role during homework, however, is to be a supervisor who monitors performance and who pro-vides frequent praise for productive behaviors.

9. **Here are the rules!** Post the ground rules for the homework ritual prominently. This should include each aspect discussed above, such as when homework is to begin, where it is to be completed, and when the Homework Assignment Sheet is to be shown to the parent. Make a game of devising a clear, meaningful poster of the ritual. Use poster board or construction paper. Change the appearance of the poster periodically.

10. **Be patient but persistent.** Stick to the homework ritual on a consistent basis, and you will soon find yourselves expending much less energy on the basics of homework.

HOMEWORK RITUAL WORKSHEET

Where?		____ Consistent place?
		____ Minimal distractions?
		____ Can I easily supervise?
When?		____ Consistent time to begin?
		____ Time limits?
		____ Homework broken into segments?
		____ Scheduled short breaks?
What?		____ Homework Assignment Sheet completed and signed by teacher?
		____ Child has materials from school?
		____ Child has supplies (e.g., pencils, paper)?

EFFECTIVE INSTRUCTIONS

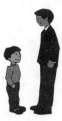

1. **Don't compete with the TV.** Instructions that you intend to give should be issued with as few distractions as possible. Therefore, make sure that your child is not distracted by the television, stereo, or video games when you issue a request.

2. **Maintain eye contact.** You are much more likely to have your child's attention if you make and keep eye contact.

3. **Keep instructions brief.** Given that children with ADHD typically have problems following directions, particularly those involving more than one step, it is important to issue instructions in simple statements. Limit them to one specific behavior at a time. *Example*: "Please put your books on the desk." *Not*: "Put your books on the desk, take out the worksheet, and do the first 10 problems."

4. **Use a neutral tone of voice.** Many children with ADHD are highly reactive to the emotional tone of instructions given by others. Consequently, such children often respond in an oppositional or hostile manner to the instruction, ignoring or not noticing the actual content of the message.

5. **Make it a statement!** In other words, an instruction should not be given as either a question or favor.

   Question: "Do you want to start homework now?"
   Favor: "Would you do me a favor and get out your homework book?"
   Statement: "Please begin your assignment now."

6. **Be reasonable**. Make your instructions reasonable and achievable. Don't set your child up to fail. Remember the saying, "Choose your battles carefully."

7. **Mean what you say and say only what you mean.** Show your child you mean what you say by issuing instructions firmly and by being *prepared to follow up* on promised consequences. Remember, actions speak louder than words, despite how loudly our words can be stated. Be patient with your child's responses as you begin to use this technique. At first children are likely to test you by displaying more noncompliant behaviors. The key reasons for this increase in undesirable behaviors are:

   a. Your child will not believe you are serious until you consistently demonstrate follow-through.
   b. Your child will not initially like your reassertion of authority.

8. **Please tell me what I just said.** Tell your child to repeat each simple instruction. This may feel awkward to you at first. However, by telling your child to repeat what you have requested, you get the benefits of:

   a. Making sure you were heard.
   b. Getting feedback as to *how* your instructions are heard. For instance, you may not realize that you

are giving multiple-step, overly complicated directions until your child attempts to repeat what you have said.

Remember to praise your child when simple instructions are correctly repeated back to you. Also praise partial correctness (e.g., "Terrific! I did say that it is time to begin, but we agreed to work on math first."). If your child does not repeat your instruction at all correctly, state it again in a calm voice, and again ask her or him to state it back to you.

9. **Have positive consequences prepared ahead of time.** State these clearly when you issue the instruction. (More on these later.) *Example*: "Bobby, if you finish these five math problems, you can pick a reward from this list."

10. **I am only going to say this once.** Make clear to your child how many times you are willing to repeat an instruction before you will enforce negative consequences. Our recommendation is to issue the direction, give your child 15 seconds to comply, issue a warning if necessary, and then within 5 additional seconds provide a consequence if your child does not comply.

USING POSITIVE REINFORCEMENT

Positive reinforcement refers to providing a consequence that makes a behavior more likely to happen again. Positive reinforcement is a very powerful tool for changing behavior and is generally preferable to punishment.

Parents often express their opinion that "my child misbehaves in order to get attention." Statements such as this reveal a common understanding that attention is a powerful reinforcer of behavior. There are many examples of how positive reinforcement plays a role in daily life. For instance, if you did not receive a paycheck for going to work and doing your job (positive reinforcement), you would probably stop going to that job. Furthermore, if your boss is someone who lets you know when you are doing a good job, you are more likely to want to work harder for that person.

A key to using positive reinforcement as a strategy for changing behavior is to selectively reinforce specific desirable behaviors and to consistently withhold reinforcement for undesirable behaviors. For example, a reward may be given for beginning homework on time, with no reward earned for beginning homework late. Using positive reinforcement makes sense, and most parents are aware of its applicability in many areas of life. However, there are often a number of challenges to consistently providing positive reinforcement with children who have ADHD.

1. **ADHD.** Children with ADHD often display more disruptive and unproductive behaviors than cooperative and responsible behaviors. Parents of children with ADHD may feel that it is difficult to find examples of cooperative behaviors to reinforce.
2. **Let sleeping dogs lie.** Many parents do not praise their child out of concern that if they do so, disruptive behaviors will soon resurface. *This concern often has a basis in fact.* The problem, however, is that when the "sleeping dog" approach is used, parents do not reinforce cooperative behavior and may end up inadvertently reinforcing undesirable actions.
3. **I object!** Sometimes parents do not feel particularly comfortable giving rewards for their children's appropriate behaviors. These objections take several forms:

   a. "I should not have to reward my child for things she should already be doing." We agree: Your child *should* already be acting appropriately. However, he or she is *not* behaving in a way that works well in your home. *Reality check: Start with where your child is, not with where you think your child should be.*
   b. "I'll go broke!" As you will see, reinforcers that do not involve money are actually preferable to ones for which you must pay. The bottom line is that you are in control of the structure of this system and should feel comfortable with it.
   c. "My child will expect to get something every time he behaves well." *First things first:* The immediate goal is to improve your child's behavior and performance. Over time you may find that you can gradually reduce the frequency of rewards and change the kinds of reinforcers you provide. For now, however, provide reinforcers very, very frequently.

d. "There's nothing my child wants," or "Something that's rewarding one week is ineffective the next week." These objections highlight the need to use variety (and mystery), particularly in dealing with a child with ADHD, when providing reinforcement. For some children it will be difficult to identify effective reinforcers. Be creative, and be sure to ask your child about what he or she may like to earn. Ask other parents as well for reinforcer ideas.

e. "This all takes too much time." As with all changes in parenting routines, the establishment of a positive reinforcement system takes some time. As it becomes routine, however, little additional time will be required.

TYPES OF POSITIVE REINFORCERS

There are four main categories of positive reinforcers. As you review these categories, you may note that your child responds well to different types of reinforcers in different situations.

1. **Sense of personal pride.** This refers to the intrinsic feelings of accomplishment an individual gets for a job well done. Although many parents believe that their child should be motivated mainly by personal pride, in many situations this type of reinforcement is not sufficient, particularly for a child with ADHD.

2. **Attention.** This pertains to becoming involved with another person in response to a particular set of behaviors. Specifically regarding a parent and child, attention can take the form of any sort of engagement with your child, in both verbal and nonverbal ways. Remember that attention can be either positive or negative. The focus here is on using positive attention. We recommend that parents use a variety of verbal and nonverbal attention reinforcers, such as: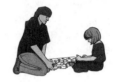

"Nice job"	"I like it when you work so hard"
"Keep up the good work"	Thumbs-up sign
Winks	Hugs
Smiles	High-fives

3. **Privileges.** Special activities that must be earned. Some examples:

Taking a trip to the park	Helping make dessert
Having a late bedtime	30 minutes of television time
30 minutes of video game	Playing a special game
Going to the movies	Spending the night with friends
Having a party	Eating out
Planting a garden	Being excused from a chore

4. **Concrete rewards.** Prizes, stickers, and tokens. Some examples:

Money	New clothes
Toys	Special snack
Tokens/points toward rewards	Select own gift

Personal pride, attention and verbal praise, and privileges are preferable to relying on the use of concrete rewards. However, it is important to recognize that concrete rewards can be very effective, and in some cases necessary, in changing and shaping behaviors.

(cont.)

REWARD MENU

Positive reinforcement systems tend to be more effective when children know ahead of time that they will have a reward menu from which to choose. Select a good time to sit down and tell your child, "We are going to start a program in which you can earn things. Let's start a list." If your child names an expensive item or time-consuming activity, you can direct the child to cut a picture of the item out of a magazine or to draw a picture of the activity. The picture can then be cut into smaller pieces. Each time the child earns a reinforcer, a part of the picture can be pasted onto a piece of paper on the refrigerator. When the picture is completed the reinforcer is earned! Also, we recommend that reinforcers be divided into:

    a. Reinforcers that can be earned on a daily basis (frequent reinforcers).
    b. Reinforcers that can be earned on a weekly basis (can also be used for bonuses).
    c. "Bigger ticket" items that can be earned from tokens or points.

VARIETY

Reward systems tend to become stale. Therefore, it is important to vary the list frequently. An element of mystery often increases a child's motivation to increase desirable behaviors. For instance, the name of a reward can be written on a piece of paper and placed in an envelope, with the envelope labeled "mystery motivator." Alternately, there can be a "grab bag" of small prizes, such as those that can be purchased at a dollar store. Some parents have also found the use of a "wheel of fortune"-type spinner or Velcro dartboard to be helpful ways of keeping mystery and variety in the reward system, with the child receiving the reinforcer that corresponds to the number that is obtained on the spinner or board.

BONUS TIME!

Your child should know that bonuses are always available for exceptionally good behavior. Many parents like to give a bonus for good *attitude*, such as cooperating and beginning work without being asked.

TOKENS AND POINTS

Giving concrete rewards or privileges to a child each time he or she is productive is usually not practical. Tokens and points, on the other hand, tend to be more practical in helping parents stick to the basic principles discussed below. Some parents keep tokens in their pocket at all times so that positive behaviors can be immediately reinforced. An additional handout will be provided that provides guidelines for using a token or point system.

FUNDAMENTAL PRINCIPLES

Many parents have previously tried some form of positive reinforcement system. However, some of the basic principles may have been omitted. We refer to the basic system as CISS-4:

    Consistency: Reward consistently for desirable behaviors.
    Immediacy: To the extent possible, give rewards immediately.
    Specificity: Be very clear about what you expect.
    Saliency: Use reinforcers that are meaningful to your child.
    4-to-1: Positive-to-negative ratio for responses.

Consistency

Easier said than done, we know, but reward systems usually do not work well when they are used inconsistently. With consistency, both you and your child will know exactly which behaviors will be responded to and in what manner. You are also likely to find that arguments and other conflicts will be reduced.

Immediacy

Immediate positive responses to productive behaviors can make a large difference. Don't delay! For tasks that are lengthy, such as homework, provide reinforcers as soon as you notice examples of productive and attentive behaviors.

Specificity

Being very specific about what you expect and what you are reinforcing is critical. Rewarding a child for "being good" can be very confusing and does not inform the child specifically what he or she has done to be reinforced. Consequently, reinforcement delivered in a nonspecific manner may not be that useful in increasing the likelihood that a child's behavior will improve. Thus, instead of saying "you earned a reward coupon for being good," you may wish to say, "you earned a reward coupon for following my directions without any reminders."

Saliency

Making sure that rewards are *meaningful* to your child seems like an obvious point. Families cannot afford to get too comfortable with reward systems, however, because what is meaningful to your child this month may not be very attractive next month. Remember that as your child becomes familiar with the system, his or her preferences for rewards will change.

4-to-1 Positive-to-Negative Ratio

We have already discussed how important and challenging it can be to get into the habit of giving positive reinforcement. There is a place for using punishment, as you will see in future sessions. However, even when punishments are introduced, it is vital that the frequency of positive reinforcers far outweigh that of punishments. Keeping a 4-to-1 ratio will make you feel more positive about managing your child's behavior, and research has shown such a ratio to be very effective. And, in turn, you will be more likely to be seen by your child as someone for whom it is good to work, a "good boss."

IMPORTANCE OF PRACTICE

At this point it is important that you use positive reinforcement extremely frequently. Pay close attention to what your child is doing, and make it a point to notice the productive and cooperative behaviors. In some families this may entail giving praise or a token for complying with such commonplace parental requests as passing the salt at the dinner table. The key point here is to make a radical shift in the ratio of positive to negative feedback you are giving to your child and to get into more positive parenting habits.

WE'VE TRIED THIS BEFORE: IT WORKS FOR A WEEK AND THEN STOPS WORKING

If you are thinking this right now, we encourage you to reread this handout and closely examine where in the CISS-4 system your previous approach may have been somewhat weak. As with the other strategies taught in this program, if you experience problems, please call us.

BE PATIENT!

Many parents report large increases in compliance almost as soon as a positive reinforcement system is begun. However, it may take a week or more of consistently using the system before you begin to notice results. With an emphasis on "catching 'em being good," though, we are confident that over time you will begin to experience changes in behavior and an improvement in your relationship with your child.

HOMEWORK REWARDS WORKSHEET

		Week of __/__/__				
# of points	Behavior	Monday	Tuesday	Wednesday	Thursday	Fri-Sat-Sun
	Bonus points for (write in):					
	Totals					

Total points for week: _____

HOMEWORK REWARDS WORKSHEET (Susan's Sample)

# of points	Behavior	Monday	Tuesday	Wednesday	Thursday	Fri-Sat-Sun
	Week of 12/5/99					
10	Homework book signed by teacher	10	10			10
5	Work area neat	5	5		5	
10	Materials ready	10			10	
15	Work started after one request		15		15	
15	Stayed on task for 10 mins.	15			15	15
10	Returned to work after breaks by one request		10			10
	Bonus points for (write in):		No reminders needed! 25			Didn't roll eyes! 10
	Totals	40	65	0	45	45

Total points for week: _190!!_

TOKEN AND POINT SYSTEM GUIDELINES

You are already familiar with some of the main categories of positive reinforcers: a sense of pride or accomplishment, verbal and nonverbal praise, privileges, and concrete reinforcers. As we have seen, reinforcement from each category can be effective for different types of tasks and situations. When attempting to improve homework performance in a child with ADHD, however, most parents find that reinforcers that are intangible and given verbally are usually not powerful enough to result in consistent gains in homework-related behaviors and performance. Establishing and using a token or point system can provide you and your child with a means of consistently and immediately reinforcing positive behaviors in a way that is simple yet meaningful. This handout summarizes the main points discussed in the Homework Success Program regarding the use of such systems. You are encouraged to refer to these guidelines from time to time as you use and revise your individualized system.

The first step is to decide whether you will use tokens or points. Older children (e.g., 10 years of age and older) and those with relatively mild ADHD may respond well to the use of points. On the other hand, younger children and those with relatively severe ADHD will often require the use of tokens. During the initial stages of your use of these reinforcement systems, do not penalize your child for undesirable behaviors by removing tokens or points. During this time "withdrawals" should take place only when your child wishes to exchange tokens or points for a concrete reinforcer or privilege.

TOKEN SYSTEM

1. **Introduce the system to your child.** Sit down with your child and discuss the system you are about to implement. Present this in a positive light, such as, "We are going to begin using a system to reward you for all the efforts you are putting in at homework time." Mention that each of the important homework behaviors will be rewarded when displayed. Have the following materials ready:

   Tokens, chips, coins, or "homework money" (see below).
   A container in which the tokens will be placed when earned.
   Cardboard or colored paper on which to tape tokens or chips (e.g., tape 1 blue, 1 red, and 1 white poker chip on the paper with their values written below them)
   Homework Rewards Worksheet

   Refer to the Homework Rewards Worksheet. Point to each behavior and tell your child that a token will be placed in the container for each behavior that is displayed. For instance, a token can be earned for beginning homework with no more than one reminder. Emphasize that bonus tokens can be earned for exceptional behaviors, such as cooperation and completing homework without arguing.

2. **Tokens and alternatives.** This handout refers to "tokens," but there are several alternatives that can be used. Alternatives to tokens include poker chips, coins, or "homework money." Homework money refers to slips of paper on which you and your child write a number of points and draw a picture. These slips can be created in increments of 1, 5, 10, and 20 "homework dollars." Likewise, you may wish to

assign values of 1, 5, and 10 points to white, red, and blue poker chips, respectively. In any case, a sample of the token or alternative that is selected should be posted near the homework location.

3. **Prepare the container.** You and your child should then decorate a token container with colorful pictures or drawings. The container and tokens will be brought out during homework time but should otherwise remain in your possession. Demonstrate for your child how the container will be used by placing a token in it for cooperative behaviors displayed while the system is being discussed.

4. **Reward menu.** A reward menu should now be created for use with this system. The first step in creating a menu is to brainstorm reinforcer ideas. Some children will volunteer primarily expensive items, which are inappropriate for daily use as reinforcers. Do not criticize your child's ideas, but if he or she suggests primarily expensive items, write them on the reward menu in a category labeled "longer term rewards." Then provide examples of reinforcers that can be earned on a short-term basis, such as a special dessert, 30 minutes of television or video game time, and exemption from doing a chore for the night. After the ideas have been generated, create a more formal-looking reward menu. You are encouraged to make the reward menu appear as attractive as possible. Many parents choose to create a reward menu that resembles a restaurant menu. Particularly at the outset, do not make the price of rewards overly expensive, or else your child may become discouraged and lose interest in the system. Here is a selection from a sample reward menu:

Reward	Price
30 minutes of television	5 chips
Trip to movies	25 chips
Weekend sleepover	100 chips

5. **Optional progress tools.** It may at times be difficult for you and your child to keep track of how many tokens have been earned, particularly if the child is seeking to earn a "big ticket" item or privilege requiring many tokens. In such cases you may wish to draw a "thermometer," which will be gradually filled in as tokens are earned. Write the name of the desired reinforcer at the top of the thermometer; when it is completely filled in the reinforcer is earned! Alternately, a picture or drawing of a desired reinforcer can be cut up into smaller "puzzle" pieces. As each piece is earned (e.g., 5 points per piece), the pieces of the puzzle are posted together until it is completed. Again, once completed the reinforcer is earned.

6. **Variety: The spice of positive reinforcement.** Be sure to include variety both in the way you *deliver* reinforcers and in the *diversity of items* on the reward menu.

Delivery of reinforcers. Short-term reinforcers, or items that can be issued very frequently, may be delivered by way of a "wheel of fortune"-type spinner, Velcro dartboard, grab bag, or "mystery motivator." Regarding the use of a spinner or dartboard, once having earned (for example) 10 points, your child may spin the wheel or toss a Velcro ball. The reinforcer that is earned will be the one on which the wheel pointer or ball lands. A grab bag can be filled with dollar-store items or with slips of paper on which you have written special activities or privileges. When using a mystery motivator, an item (or slip of paper with the item or privilege written on it) is placed in an envelope. The outside of the envelope may have a question mark written on it. The envelope should be prominently placed for the child to see. It has been found that the element of surprise in all of the suggested delivery methods described above tends to increase children's interest in, and enjoyment of, positive reinforcement systems.

Variety of reinforcers. It is important that the reward menu be periodically revised to ensure that only effective reinforcers are on the list. You are aware that your child's interests change over time. Thus an item or privilege that may be a powerful reinforcer when you initially use your system may lose its effectiveness over time in promoting productive behaviors. Be sure to review the reward menu with your child on a monthly basis to add and delete items as indicated.

7. **"Dad, please give me the reward now! I promise I'll finish my work!"** Some children will attempt to bargain with parents, saying that they will be productive in the future if they can get a reinforcer im-

(cont.)

mediately. Many parents find this to be a situation in which they are tempted to defer to the child's wishes. It is important, however, that reinforcers be delivered only after the target behaviors have been displayed. Such an approach ensures consistency and structure in your reinforcement system.

8. **How about when a reinforcer has not been earned?** If a reinforcer is not earned, do not criticize your child. Merely express your hope that she or he will earn the reinforcer during the next homework session, and refer to the Homework Rewards Worksheet as a reminder of which behaviors need to be displayed at that time.

9. **Tip the scales toward success!** Your positive reinforcement system should be devised so that your child earns a reinforcer about 80% of the time. This is important because overly stringent standards may very well discourage your child and lead to conflict and frustration. On the other hand, if your child earns reinforcers nearly 100% of the time, there is little incentive for behavior changes.

10. **Be patient.** Some children may oppose the use of a positive reinforcement system during homework time, particularly in the initial stages of using the system. Presenting the system in a positive manner should help reduce such opposition. Particularly if your child does not earn reinforcers immediately, you should persist with the program, tip the scales toward success, and remind yourself to be patient. Most children ultimately find the experience to be a positive and enjoyable one.

POINT SYSTEM

Most of the guidelines pertaining to token systems are also appropriate when using a point system. There are a few special considerations, however.

1. **The "bankbook."** Parents should create a "bankbook" when planning a point system for homework time. There should be columns for date, "deposit" of points, "withdrawal," and balance. You may wish to label the front of this simply as "Homework Bankbook," or use a label suggested by your child.

2. **Open for business!** As with token containers, a point-system bankbook should be kept in your possession except during homework time. In order to jump-start the system, you may wish to place 100 points (for example) in the account as a reward to your child for cooperation during the initial discussion of the point system. At the outset of homework time, display the bankbook in front of your child and remind him or her about the current balance.

3. **Deposits and withdrawals.** Using a tool such as the Homework Rewards Worksheet (see Handout 11), keep track of points earned during homework. When homework is completed, you should supervise your child while she or he enters points earned in the "deposit" column of bankbook. Provide similar supervision when points are withdrawn for use in purchasing reinforcers from the reward menu.

OTHER CONSIDERATIONS

Some parents may have reservations about particular aspects of a token or point system or may object to using such a system at all. Refer to the handout on positive reinforcement in order to address common concerns of parents, such as beliefs regarding "bribery" and the amount of time reinforcement systems consume. Note that if you have other children who are also in elementary school, they may wish to have their own token or point systems for homework, particularly once they notice that their brother or sister is earning reinforcers for productive and cooperative behaviors during homework. In such cases, you are encouraged to devise a token or point system that is appropriate to the other children's needs and developmental level.

MANAGING TIME AND GOAL SETTING

The first key to effective time management and goal setting is to look closely and honestly at where your child and you are at this point. Review your progress regarding giving effective instructions: Be clear, direct, specific, and consistent with consequences. Keep up the positive reinforcement system. Give yourself some praise for your efforts and some to your child for his or her efforts. *It will be important to maintain your daily logs each day, including on-task time and total amount of time spent on homework, in order to monitor progress.*

1. **Dear diary . . .** Your daily logs should include a daily estimate of the length of time your child was able to remain on task.
2. **OK, break it up!** Homework should be subdivided into smaller units of relatively equal length. You can divide homework by subject area and (if homework for a particular subject is lengthy) according to the amount of work required for each subject. Remember to keep in mind your child's unique attention span. Be generous regarding how long you think each subunit should take for your child to complete. We have found that a simple formula for subunit length is *about 3 minutes for each grade level.* For instance, a fourth-grader may have subunits of 12 minutes each.
3. **Break it up?** By segmenting assignments in this manner, your child is more likely to be able to sustain attention to the particular subunit. Note that the end of each subunit is an opportunity to provide a quick yet meaningful positive reinforcer (e.g., praise, small reward, or points toward a privilege), although (as described in the step-by-step guidelines below) it is important that you give your child specific verbal praise while he or she is actually working.
4. **Supervisor and tutor.** The distinction between your roles as supervisor and tutor has been previously discussed. This point in the program is a particularly crucial time to remind yourself of this distinction. Your *primary* role is to supervise your child's homework. Your role as *tutor* should only come into play in making sure, at the outset, that your child understands the directions and, at the conclusion of homework for a particular subject, to *briefly* review the work.
5. **Let's be realistic.** Teachers occasionally report to us that a particular child's rate of homework completion and accuracy is about 100%. These children are often the ones who spend 4 hours or more on homework, with frustrated parents becoming accustomed to a pattern of standing over the child until work is done. Although this pattern can temporarily address a parent's fears of a child "falling behind," the strain on the parent–child relationship can be quite severe. We have a tool. . . .
6. **Goal-Setting Tool (GST).** Time limits are now to be used in a very systematic fashion. This system may at first seem intimidating. However, we have found that the GST can be very effective when used consistently and correctly. It is recommended that you and your child learn how to use it in steps. These steps, when taken one at a time, will help to more easily make the GST a part of your homework routine. We will provide you with a demonstration regarding how to use the GST and will also give assistance to you as you practice its use. Please be sure to ask questions as they arise. You may also need to refer to the GST worksheet attached to this handout.

USING THE GOAL-SETTING TOOL

1. **Decide ahead of time what the reward will be when goals are met.** Present this as an opportunity to earn something positive. Decide how many points are needed to earn the reward, and follow the GST guidelines for distributing points after each subunit of work. Be clear about what you expect, including how many points are required for the reward.

2. **Break up the assignment into subunits**, as noted above. This will take some practice and will initially seem as if you are actually increasing homework time. As the GST becomes a part of the daily routine, you will begin to see it providing clear expectations and structure for your child. Consistent use of the GST should also ultimately be associated with significant reductions in homework time and with noticeable increases in productivity.

3. **Set time limits.** Decide how much time your child will be permitted for each subunit. As noted, about 3 minutes for each grade level is advised. However, feel free to adjust this time limit in order to ensure success at least 80% of the time. Write this in under "Time" in Step 1 of the GST.

4. **Set completion goals.** For each subunit, ask your child how many of the problems he or she thinks can be completed in the time limit. This is another important opportunity for you and your child to improve your negotiating skills. Based on your experience supervising homework, you may know that your child is typically able to complete 5 problems in this period. However, do not be surprised if your child believes that 10 is a realistic goal. In such cases, you are encouraged to compromise on a goal of 7 or 8. Write that in for the "# Items completed" in Step 1 of the GST.

5. **Set accuracy goals.** Having set a completion goal, the next step is to negotiate the *accuracy goal* with your child. From the above example, the two of you may decide that 5 correct answers is a reasonable goal. It is important that you guide your child to set goals that will ensure that he or she succeeds at least 80% of the time. Write the accuracy goal in the "# Items correct" slot in Step 1 of the GST.

6. **Make sure your child understands the directions.** Remember that during the time that your child is working on each subunit, you will be providing verbal praise for on-task behaviors and will be keeping an eye on the clock. In other words, you will be engaging in supervision activities. It is very important that you make sure your child understands what to do before beginning each subunit of work.

7. **Get ready!** Set the *countdown timer.* Instruct your child that he or she is to keep working during this time and that you will be checking to make sure that homework is being completed.

8. **Provide verbal praise.** While your child is working, it is important that you provide verbal praise for on-task behaviors and productive work. Remember to be specific. Particularly while you are both getting used to using the GST, a general guideline is to provide verbal praise about two to three times per subunit. Do not respond to requests for assistance with the work during this time. If such a request is made, tell your child to keep working and that you will give assistance when the time limit is up.

9. **Direct child to evaluate work.** At the end of the time limit, compliment your child for the work that was completed. Then direct your child to Step 2 of the GST. Have your child write in the appropriate slots how many items she or he completed and how many he or she thinks are correct. You should then check your child's work to make sure that accurate information has been entered in Step 2.

10. **Evaluate completion.** In Step 3 of the GST, place a check mark in the appropriate slot, depending on whether your child exceeded the completion goal, met the goal, or did not meet the goal.

11. **Evaluate accuracy.** Follow the same procedures for Step 4 as for Step 3, this time focusing on *accuracy.* Indicate how your child fared relative to the accuracy goals.

12. **Count up total points.** In Step 5 of the GST, write in points earned based on what was noted for Steps 3 and 4. Be sure to praise your child's efforts regardless of whether a reinforcer has been earned.

13. **Provide rewards!** At the end of homework, be sure to give the reinforcer if it has been earned. Remember that if your child is not succeeding at least 80% of the time, you may need to adjust the goals.

Remember, once the subunit is over, *do not redo it, even if there are inaccuracies.* Move on. If your child has not met the goal, do not belabor the point. Eventually you should find that not earning the reward motivates your child in the future.

GOAL-SETTING TOOL

Date: _____

Step 1. What is my goal?

# items completed	_____
# items correct	_____
Time	_____

Step 2. How did I do?

# items completed	_____
# items correct	_____

Step 3. Did I reach my completion goal? (Circle one)

	Points
Yes, far above goal	2
Yes, I met my goal	1
No, goal not met	0

Step 4. Did I reach my correctness goal? (Circle one)

	Points
Yes, far above goal	2
Yes, I met the goal	1
No, goal not met	0

Step 5. Total points!

_____ + _____ = _____
Completion   Correctness   Total points
(from Step 3)   (from Step 4)

____ (Check here after giving praise for effort.)

GOAL-SETTING TOOL: SUMMARY WORKSHEET

Date: _____

Subject: _____

Goals: Items completed: _____ Items correct: _____ Time: _____

Performance: Items completed: _____ Items correct: _____ Time: _____

Did I reach my completion goal? (*Circle one*): 2 (Far above goal) 1 (Met goal) 0 (Goal not met)

Did I reach my correctness goal? (*Circle one*): 2 (Far above goal) 1 (Met goal) 0 (Goal not met)

Total points _____ + _____ = _____
$\quad\quad\quad\quad$ Completion $\quad\quad\quad\quad$ Correctness $\quad\quad\quad\quad$ Total points

___ (Check here after giving praise for effort)

Subject: _____

Goals: Items completed: ___ Items correct: ___ Time: ___

Performance: Items completed: ___ Items correct: ___ Time: ___

Did I reach my completion goal? (*Circle one*): 2 (Far above goal) 1 (Met goal) 0 (Goal not met)

Did I reach my correctness goal? (*Circle one*): 2 (Far above goal) 1 (Met goal) 0 (Goal not met)

Total points _____ + _____ = _____
$\quad\quad\quad\quad$ Completion $\quad\quad\quad\quad$ Correctness $\quad\quad\quad\quad$ Total points

___ (Check here after giving praise for effort)

Subject: _____

Goals: Items completed: ___ Items correct: ___ Time: ___

Performance: Items completed: ___ Items correct: ___ Time: ___

Did I reach my completion goal? (*Circle one*): 2 (Far above goal) 1 (Met goal) 0 (Goal not met)

Did I reach my correctness goal? (*Circle one*): 2 (Far above goal) 1 (Met goal) 0 (Goal not met)

Total points _____ + _____ = _____
$\quad\quad\quad\quad$ Completion $\quad\quad\quad\quad$ Correctness $\quad\quad\quad\quad$ Total points

___ (Check here after giving verbal for effort)

USING PUNISHMENT SUCCESSFULLY

Due to the disruptive and unproductive behaviors displayed by most children with ADHD, many parents are well acquainted with procedures such as time-out, removal of privileges, and other punishments. We are often told by parents that "no discipline seems to work." Indeed, with children who have ADHD and are defiant toward their parents, punishment frequently does not have much of an effect on child behavior.

Punishment can be an effective disciplinary strategy, but it is vital that it be used *strategically.* When children become accustomed to receiving large doses of criticism and punishments, they often give up easily when they are unsure if they will succeed. Therefore, the emphasis in any sound behavioral program should remain on incentives and positive reinforcers. On the other hand, with children who have impulse control difficulties, systems that *only* include positive reinforcement are often not adequate.

1. **Know yourself.** Observe your reactions when you deliver punishment to your child. The key word is *observe*, not judge. Your emotional responses to your child's misbehavior are critical. If you are harsh and highly emotional, your child's misbehavior may escalate. If you are firm and under control, on the other hand, you will be more successful in managing misbehavior.

2. **Key word: *Strategic.*** Remember, when you use punishments, you must remain in control of the situation. Therefore, use punishment sparingly until you are comfortable with the consistency and structure of your positive reinforcement system for homework.

3. **Keep a 4-to-1 ratio.** That is, make sure that the amount of positive reinforcement you use is at least four times the amount of punishment. This approach will help to prevent unintended side effects, such as discouragement, anger, and aggressiveness.

4. **Mean what you say, and say what you mean.** Be clear and firm in delivering punishments. Don't tell your child that she or he will be grounded for 6 months unless you are interested in giving *yourself* some serious punishment. Be ready to back up what you say with a consequence.

5. **Choose *correction* whenever possible.** Correction offered verbally and nonverbally can be an effective form of punishment. When giving correction, state what the child *should* do (e.g., "You are supposed to begin work *now*."), not what the child should *not* do (e.g., "Stop daydreaming and wasting time!").

6. **Provide correction *immediately.*** The goal is to respond to your child as soon as possible after misbehavior occurs. We acknowledge that responding immediately is not always possible, but it should be the goal and standard practice.

7. **Be *specific.*** Specify the behavior that the child needs to improve (e.g., "You need to pay attention to your work"). Avoid vague statements (e.g., "You're doing badly").

(cont.)

---

8. **Keep your corrections *simple* and *brief*.** Correction is useful if it is stated clearly and very briefly.

9. **Be firm, but not harsh.** State the correction in a firm manner that indicates you are serious about what you are saying. Avoid asking questions (e.g., "Would you mind getting back to work?").

10. **Response cost.** Response cost is a particularly useful technique for children with ADHD. Response cost refers to the removal of positive reinforcers, such as points, privileges, or rewards. Include response cost in your token reinforcement system. For example, your child can earn points for productive work but can lose points for hitting a sibling or for leaving the homework location. However, be sure to keep in mind the 4-to-1 positive–negative ratio.

11. **Time-out.** Time-out usually is effective in managing behavior. However, we do not recommend this strategy in managing homework problems because time-out can reinforce children by getting them out of doing homework.

12. **Use of punishment in nonhomework situations.** Over time you may wish to apply these punishment strategies in situations besides homework. However, make sure that you use the CISS-4 principles and that punishment does not become the primary behavior management technique. Keeping these points in mind will help to prevent "backsliding" into an overly punitive system.

13. **Remember CISS-4.** Remember, the basics are consistency, immediacy, specificity, saliency (meaningfulness), and a 4-to-1 positive-to-negative ratio.

MAINTAINING SUCCESS
AND ANTICIPATING FUTURE PROBLEMS

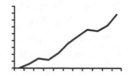

Many images could be used to describe the challenge of successfully managing your child's homework. At first it can seem like a juggling act, with parents struggling to use all of the different components of Homework Success: the homework ritual, effective instructions, positive reinforcement, the A-B-C Worksheets, the Goal-Setting Tool, and strategic use of punishment. Perhaps even at this time, it is not clear how these different parts fit together. Our hope is that these components are at least starting to become part of your routine. And as you integrate the parts, what you should experience is an improvement of your parent–child relationship and more homework success.

It may be most appropriate to picture all of these elements put together like a *symphony*. And like all symphony conductors, you will have to continue to pay attention to what is going on around you and make adjustments as needed. *Remember: It is an ongoing process.* At times the strategies will work nicely together, and your child will respond productively and cooperatively. At other times you may overemphasize one element (e.g., punishment) and need to accentuate the importance of another element (e.g., positive reinforcement).

So here's our "handbook" on putting it all together and looking to the future.

1. **Some progress? Any progress?** Perhaps you are fairly pleased with the progress you and your child have made over the course of this program. Or maybe you are wondering if you've actually made progress at all. It is our experience that most parents are somewhere in between feeling on top of the world about homework and feeling totally discouraged. In other words, at this point in the program most parents report that they have made significant gains but would still like to improve homework time. Even if you are not particularly satisfied with your progress, a close look at where you are should reveal at least *some* changes for the better.

   In order to keep steady regarding the progress you have made, it is helpful to assess your knowledge and experiences regarding each component of the program.

2. **Remember the relation between ADHD and homework.** The inattention, impulsivity, and (often) hyperactivity associated with ADHD can account for many homework problems. When you refer back to Handout 3 (ADHD: Basic Facts) and Handout 4 (Some Ways ADHD Is Related to Homework Problems), you will be reminded that ADHD is not caused by faulty parenting. Children who by nature are forgetful will have problems completing their homework assignment books, remembering to bring home the books needed for homework, and consistently beginning work on time. Likewise, children who are distractible tend to have particular problems remaining on task during homework time. Keep in mind that homework problems are very, very common among children with ADHD and that homework success requires specialized techniques and strategies.

3. **Follow the A-B-Cs.** When a particular behavior is displayed by a child, he or she is usually getting something rewarding out of it or is avoiding an unpleasant situation. Antecedents (A's) are what comes first. Examples include the Homework Ritual and how instructions are given. The behaviors (B's) of interest

(cont.)

are what follow the A's. Consequences (C's) are responses to specific behaviors. Examples of consequences include ignoring inappropriate behaviors and praising compliance with commands. We strongly encourage an approach to behavior management that continues to look closely at the A-B-C's.

4. **Use a Homework Ritual.** By now each of you should have a consistent homework ritual. Refer as needed to Handout 7 (Establishing the Homework Ritual) and Handout 8 (Homework Ritual Worksheet) to make sure that the *where, when,* and *what* of homework are consistent and clear. Set up the homework environment in such a way that your child is likely to be productive and cooperative.

5. **Give effective instructions.** Giving instructions properly is a necessary step in improving your child's behavior. Refer to Handout 9 (Effective Instructions) and review these tips:

   Don't compete with the TV.
   Maintain eye contact.
   State instructions briefly.
   Make it a statement.
   Be reasonable.
   Be prepared with consequences.
   Mean what you say.

6. **Stay positive!** Refer to Handout 10 (Using Positive Reinforcement) to review the basic principles of positive reinforcement. Remember how powerful your attention is, so use it strategically. Be patient, look for productive behavior, and reinforce it when you see it.

7. **Keep the token or point system going.** Handouts 11 (Homework Rewards Worksheet) and 12 (Token and Point System Guidelines) can be used as tools for strengthening the positive reinforcement you provide. When used consistently, these systems should be associated with increased productivity and cooperation.

8. **Remember CISS-4.** Have we mentioned CISS-4? You may be tired of hearing this by now, but it is important to remember these basic principles:

   Consistency is a cornerstone of behavior management. Your child must know what is acceptable and what is unacceptable. Provide positive reinforcement for desired behaviors and withhold reinforcement for undesirable behaviors. Follow these guidelines as often as you can.

   Immediacy is also important. Administer consequences as soon as you can after a targeted behavior is displayed.

   Specificity pertains to making it clear what will be rewarded or punished and being precise in your responses.

   Saliency refers to the meaningfulness of behavioral consequences. Reinforcers must be valuable to the child in order for them to be effective. Remember that what is salient one week may not mean much to your child in a month or two. So be sure to keep your reward menus fresh and interesting.

   4-to-1 refers to maintaining a ratio of 4 positive reinforcers to 1 punishment. Don't lose sight of this ratio! Your relationship with your child will benefit and behavioral improvements will be more consistent with a predominantly positive approach.

9. **Have a goal in mind.** Keep using the Goal-Setting Tool. Refer to Handout 13 (Managing Time and Goal Setting) for strategies about how to use this technique. These include segmenting work into subunits of reasonable length, setting realistic goals for completion and accuracy, evaluating performance in relation to goals, and providing reinforcement for achieving goals.

10. **Use punishment sparingly and strategically.** Refer to Handout 15 (Using Punishment Successfully) to remind yourself how to use punishment. If you find that you are slipping back into relying excessively on punishment, stop and get that positive-to-negative ratio back up to 4-to-1.

11. **Congratulate yourself!** You have probably learned some new principles to guide you during homework time. In this short program you have been asked to alter many well-established patterns of parenting. If you haven't reached perfection yet, don't worry. If you consistently use the principles outlined in the Homework Success Program, things should continue to move in a positive direction. Take time to

applaud yourself and your child for the efforts you have made, the progress you have displayed, and the strategies you have mastered to meet future challenges.

12. **Now what?** It is important that you and your child attend the booster session. At that time we will review how homework time has proceeded during the intervening weeks. Your child will also receive a diploma for graduating from the Homework Success Program. The booster session will be an opportunity for us to assist you with troubleshooting old problems that have reappeared and new ones that may have surfaced. The following is a review of some possible problems you may encounter:

   a. **The Blame Game.** The Blame Game is an old nemesis. It is easy for parents to forget that no one is necessarily at fault when behavioral problems appear. As discussed in this program, ADHD is related to numerous compliance problems, particularly regarding high-demand situations such as homework. If you find yourself falling into the blame trap, take a deep breath, forgive yourself and your child, and review what you have learned here.

   b. **"The devil whispered in my ear."** When you consistently experience progress in your child's behavior, you may have the thought that "my child must be cured." Remember, the focus of this program has been on managing behavior, not curing it. So don't be discouraged if problems reappear. You are now in a better position to navigate the ups and downs of problem behaviors related to ADHD.

   c. **"We kept it up for awhile then it kind of faded away."** Don't let this happen to you. Perhaps the most common pitfall once a program ends is to slack off on using the strategies. Remember that you and your child did not change magically. Maintaining progress will only occur through continued hard work.

   d. **"Now she wants to be rewarded for everything."** Remember that verbal praise and attention to positive behaviors are preferred responses. Effective behavioral approaches tend to gradually withdraw reinforcers as the desirable behaviors become more habitual for a child. One way to accomplish this is to provide concrete reinforcers less often. If you are using a token or point system, over time your child may need to earn more tokens or points in order to obtain reinforcers.

   e. **"It's hard to stay positive."** Some parents report that they have a difficult time remaining positive during homework time, even after completion of this program. We recommend that you keep a "recipe card" that outlines the CISS-4 principles, and have it with you during homework time. If you find yourself backsliding into giving too many punishments, keep a tally of the number of times you are giving positive reinforcement versus punishment. Increasing your self-awareness in this manner will help to change your own behavior.

   f. **"I can't seem to figure out why he does what he does."** Remember, most behaviors can be traced to getting something that is rewarding (even if it is a reprimand from a parent), or avoiding an unpleasant situation (such as beginning homework). Keep using the A-B-C worksheets to help you identify what may be sustaining a particular behavior.

   g. **"Nothing is rewarding."** We occasionally encounter children who do not respond to typical reinforcers. Parents of such children need to work harder than other parents to identify effective rewards. Of course, you are encouraged to include your child in structuring and revising the reward menu. Be creative: Ask other parents, attend a local CHADD meeting (800-233-4050), surf the Internet (the local librarian can help with this), talk with your child's psychologist, and talk with your child's teacher. You are particularly encouraged to talk with a psychologist if your child's lack of response to rewards seems to be related to depressed mood.

   h. **"Talk with my child's teacher?"** Most parents find it helpful to be in regular contact with their child's teacher. Such an approach has many potential benefits, including increasing home–school consistency, receiving timely feedback regarding your child's progress, and increasing parental involvement in learning.

   i. **"Where the heck did this come from?"** Some problems will arise that you simply cannot anticipate. From time to time you will encounter new and "interesting" problems. However, the principles you have learned in this program should serve as guidelines for meeting unanticipated challenges.

13. **Now go treat yourself to a reward.** when the session is over, and we'll see you at the booster session. Please call if needed during the interim.

RESOURCES

There are many resources for families who are coping with ADHD and homework problems. This handout lists some of the books and other resources that families have found useful.

BOOKS FOR PARENTS

Anesko, K. M., & Levine, F. M. (1987). *Winning the homework war.* New York: Simon & Schuster.

Barkley, R. (2000). *Taking charge of ADHD: The complete, authoritative guide for parents* (rev. ed.). New York: Guilford Press.

Flick, G. (1996). *Power parenting for children with ADD/ADHD.* West Nyack, NY: Center for Applied Research in Education.

Fowler, M. (1990). *Maybe you know my kid: A parent's guide to identifying, understanding, and helping your child with ADHD.* New York: Birchland.

Gordon, M. (1990). *ADHD/hyperactivity: A consumer's guide.* New York: GSI.

Markova, D., & Powell, A. R. (1998). *Learning unlimited: Using homework to engage your child's natural style of intelligence.* Berkeley, CA: Conari Press.

Parker, H. (1998). *The ADD hyperactivity workbook for parents, teachers, and kids* (2nd ed.). Plantation, FL: Impact.

Radencich, M. C., & Schumm, J. S. (1997). *How to help your child with homework* (2nd ed.). Minneapolis, MN: Free Spirit.

Zentall, S. S., & Goldstein, S. (1999). *Seven steps to homework success: A family guide for solving common homework problems.* Plantation, FL: Specialty Press.

BOOKS FOR CHILDREN

Gordon, M. (1991). *Jumpin' Johnny get back to work: A child's guide to ADHD/hyperactivity.* DeWitt, NY: GSI.

Quinn, P. O., & Stern, J. (1991). *Putting on the brakes.* New York: Magination.

Also: Parents are encouraged to join, and to participate in, a support/educational organization for families of persons with ADHD. Examples include Children and Adults with Attention Deficit Disorders (CHADD; 800-233-4050) and the Attention Deficit Disorder Advocacy Group (ADDAG; 303-690-7548).

The ADD Warehouse can send you a free catalog of books, videos, and other resources (800-ADD-WARE; www.addwarehouse.com).

Finally: As Doctor Spock said, "You know more than you think you do." However, professional support is also important at times. Work closely with your child's psychologist, physician, and school personnel to continue progress and obtain referrals for professional assistance as needed.

All of the members of the Homework Success Program wish you and your family good fortune in your endeavors!!!!

Materials for Child Group

CHILDREN'S INTERVENTION RATING PROFILE

INSTRUCTIONS

- Your group leader will read each sentence to you.
- Think about the past couple of weeks as you choose your answer.
- If you *Agree* with the sentence, circle "1" for *Yes*. If you are *Not sure* about the sentence, circle "2" for *Not sure*. If you *Disagree* with the sentence, circle "3" for *No*.
- There are no right or wrong answers. Only you can tell us what you think about this group.

		Yes 1	Not sure 2	No 3
1.	My group leader was fair.	1	2	3
2.	My group leader was too mean.	1	2	3
3.	My friends teased me because I come to this group each week.	1	2	3
4.	Other things could help me more than this group.	1	2	3
5.	This group would be good for my friends in school.	1	2	3
6.	I like coming to this group each week.	1	2	3
7.	I think that coming to this group helps me do better in school.	1	2	3

CARDS FOR THE CONCENTRATION GAME

QUESTION CARDS FOR SESSION 1: EXAMPLES

Concentration Name one problem you have when you do your homework.	*Concentration* What do you think your parents find hard about your homework?	*Concentration* Name one thing your parents can do to make your homework easier.

Concentration Name one thing that you can do to make homework easier for yourself.	*Concentration* How can you make your homework fun?

QUESTION CARDS FOR SESSION 5: EXAMPLES

Concentration What do your parents do when you pay attention and work hard while you are completing your homework?	*Concentration* What do your parents do when you do not work hard during homework time?	*Concentration* What do your parents do when you talk too much, argue, or get out of your chair during homework time?
Concentration How would you feel about losing points for disruptive homework behavior?	*Concentration* Are there some behaviors that you think your parents should punish?	*Concentration* What are some fair ways for your parents to punish you?

PICTURE PAIR CARDS

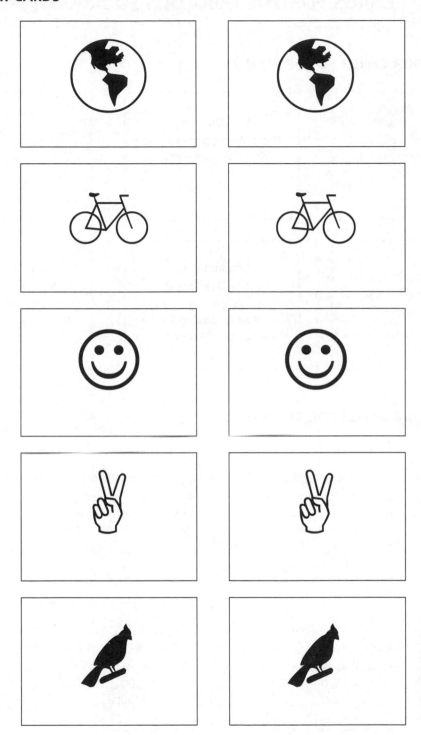

CARDS FOR THE FABULOUS FOUR GAME

FABULOUS FOUR CARDS FOR SESSION 2

Fabulous Four Name four good places to do your homework.	*Fabulous Four* Name four bad places to do your homework.	*Fabulous Four* Name four materials that you need to have with you when you do your homework.
Fabulous Four Name four good times to do your homework.	*Fabulous Four* Name four things that you do when you are tired or frustrated from doing your homework.	*Fabulous Four* Name four rewards you would like to receive when you complete your homework.

FABULOUS FOUR CARDS FOR SESSION 4

Fabulous Four Name four rewards you have received for doing your homework.	*Fabulous Four* Name four rewards you would like to receive for doing your homework.
Fabulous Four Name four things that you do that will earn you rewards for homework.	*Fabulous Four* Name four things that you do during homework that will <u>not earn you rewards.</u>

References

Abidin, R. R. (1995). *Parenting Stress Index Manual.* Charlottesville, VA: Pediatric Psychology Press.

Abikoff, H., Gittelman-Klein, R., & Klein, D. (1977). Validation of a classroom observation code for hyperactive children. *Journal of Consulting and Clinical Psychology, 45,* 772–783.

Achenbach, T. M. (1991a). *Manual for the Child Behavior Checklist/4–18 and 1991 Profile.* Burlington: University of Vermont Department of Psychiatry.

Achenbach, T. M. (1991b). *Manual for the Teacher's Report Form and 1991 Profile.* Burlington: University of Vermont Department of Psychiatry.

Aman, M. G., & Wolford, P. L. (1995). Consumer satisfaction with involvement in drug research: A social validity study. *Journal of the American Academy of Child and Adolescent Psychiatry, 34,* 940–945.

American Psychiatric Association. (1994). *Diagnostic and statistical manual of mental disorders* (4th ed.). Washington, DC: Author.

Anastasi, A., & Urbina, S. (1997). *Psychological testing* (7th ed.). Upper Saddle River, NJ: Prentice-Hall.

Anastopoulos, A. D., Shelton, T., DuPaul, G. J., & Guevremont, D. C. (1993). Parent training for attention deficit hyperactivity disorder: Its impact on parent functioning. *Journal of Abnormal Child Psychology, 21,* 581–596.

Anesko, K. M., & Levine, F. M. (1987). *Winning the homework war.* New York: Simon & Schuster.

Anesko, K. M., & O'Leary, S. G. (1982). The effectiveness of brief parent training for the management of children's homework problems. *Child and Family Behavior Therapy, 4,* 113–126.

Anesko, K. M., Schoiock, G., Ramirez, R., & Levine, F. M. (1987). The Homework Problem Checklist: Assessing children's homework difficulties. *Behavioral Assessment, 9,* 179–185.

Barkley, R. A. (1991). *Attention-deficit hyperactivity disorder: A clinical workbook.* New York: Guilford Press.

Barkley, R. A. (1997). *Defiant children* (2nd ed.): *A clinician's manual for assessment and parent training.* New York: Guilford Press.

Barkley, R. A. (1998). *Attention-deficit hyperactivity disorder: A handbook for diagnosis and treatment* (2nd ed.). New York: Guilford Press.

Barkley, R. A., McMurray, M. B., Edelbrock, C. S., & Robbins, K. (1990). The side effects of Ritalin: A systematic placebo controlled evaluation of two doses. *Pediatrics, 86,* 184–192.

Bennett, D. S., Power, T. J., Rostain, A. L., & Carr, D. E. (1996). Parent acceptability and feasibility of ADHD interventions: Assessment, correlates, and predictive validity. *Journal of Pediatric Psychology, 21,* 643–657.

Bernard, H. S., & MacKenzie, K. R. (Eds.). (1994). *Basics of group psychotherapy.* New York: Guilford Press.

Biederman, J., Newcorn, J., & Sprich, S. (1991). Comorbidity of attention deficit hyperactivity disorder with conduct, depressive, anxiety, and other disorders. *American Journal of Psychiatry, 148,* 564–577.

Black, M. M., & Krishnakumar, A. (1998). Children in low-income, urban settings: Interventions to promote mental health and well-being. *American Psychologist, 53,* 635–646.

Brown, R. T., Borden, K. A., Wynne, M. E., Spunt, A. L., & Clingerman, S. R. (1987). Compliance with pharmacological and cognitive treatments for attention deficit disorder. *Journal of the American Academy of Child and Adolescent Psychiatry, 26,* 521–526.

Brown, R. T., & Sawyer, M. G. (1998). *Medications for school-age children: Effects on learning and behavior.* New York: Guilford Press.

Buck, G. H., Bursuck, W. D., Polloway, E. A., Nelson, J., Jayanthi, M. J., & Whitehouse, F. A. (1996). Homework-related communication problems: Perspectives of special educators. *Journal of Emotional and Behavioral Disorders, 4,* 105–113.

Canter, L., & Hausner, D. (1987). *Homework without tears: A parent guide for motivating children to do homework and succeed in school.* New York: Harper & Row.

Christenson, S. L., Rounds, T., & Franklin, M. J. (1992). Home–school collaboration: Effects, issues, and opportunities. In S. L. Christenson & J. C. Conoley (Eds.), *Home–school collaboration: Enhancing children's academic and social competence.* Silver Spring, MD: National Association of School Psychologists.

Comer, J. P., & Haynes, N. M. (1991). Parent involvement in the schools: An ecological approach. *Elementary School Journal, 91,* 271–277.

Conners, C. K. (1997). *The Conners Rating Scales–Revised.* North Tonowanda, NY: Multi-Health Systems.

Cooper, H. (1989). *Homework.* White Plains, NY: Longman.

Cooper, H., Lindsay, J. J., Nye, B., & Greathouse, S. (1998). Relationships among attitudes about homework, amount of homework assigned and completed, and student achievement. *Journal of Educational Psychology, 90*(1), 70–83.

Cunningham, C. E., Bremner, R., & Boyle, M. (1995). Large group community-based parenting programs for families of preschoolers at risk for disruptive behaviour disorders: Utilization, cost effectiveness, and outcome. *Journal of Child Psychology and Psychiatry, 36,* 1141–1159.

Cunningham, C. E., & Cunningham, L. J. (1998). Student-mediated conflict resolution programs. In R. A. Barkley, *Attention-deficit hyperactivity disorder: A handbook for diagnosis and treatment* (2nd ed.). New York: Guilford Press.

Curran, D. (1989). *Working with parents.* Circle Pines, MN: American Guidance Service.

Daniel, S., Power, T. J., Karustis, J. L., & Leff, S. S. (1999, November). *Parent-mediated homework intervention for children with ADHD: Its impact on parent–child relationships and parenting stress.* Poster session presented at the annual meeting of the Association for Advancement of Behavior Therapy, Toronto, Ontario, Canada.

Dowrick, P. W., Power, T. J., Manz, P. H., Ginsburg-Block, M., Leff, S. S., & Kim-Rupnow, S. (in press). Community responsiveness: Examples from under-resourced urban schools. *Journal of Prevention and Intervention in the Community.*

Dryfoos, J. G. (1994). *Full-service schools: A revolution in health and social services for children, youth, and families.* San Francisco, CA: Jossey-Bass.

Dubey, D. R., O'Leary, S. G., & Kaufman, K. F. (1983). Training parents of hyperactive children in child management: A comparative outcome study. *Journal of Abnormal Child Psychology, 11,* 229–246.

Dumas, J. E., & Wahler, R. G. (1983). Predictors of treatment outcome in parent training: Mother insularity and socioeconomic disadvantage. *Behavioral Assessment, 5,* 301–313.

DuPaul, G. J., Barkley, R. A., & Connor, D. F. (1998). Stimulants. In R. A. Barkley, *Attention-deficit hyperactivity disorder: A handbook for diagnosis and treatment* (2nd ed.). New York: Guilford Press.

DuPaul, G. J., Eckert, T. L., & McGoey, K. E. (1997). Interventions for students with attention-deficit/hyperactivity disorder: One size does not fit all. *School Psychology Review, 26,* 369–381.

DuPaul, G. J., & Ervin, R. A. (1996). Functional assessment of behaviors related to attention-deficit hyperactivity disorder: Linking assessment to intervention design. *Behavior Therapy, 27,* 601–622.

DuPaul, G. J., & Power, T. J. (2000). Educational interventions for children with attention deficit disorders. In T. E. Brown (Ed.), *Attention deficit disorders and comorbidities in children, adolescents, and adults* (pp. 607–636). Washington, DC: American Psychiatric Press.

DuPaul, G. J., Power, T. J., Anastopoulos, A. D., & Reid, R. (1998). *ADHD Rating Scale–IV: Checklists, norms, and clinical interpretation.* New York: Guilford Press.

DuPaul, G. J., & Rapport, M. D. (1993). Does methylphenidate normalize the classroom performance of children with attention deficit disorder? *Journal of the American Academy of Child and Adolescent Psychiatry, 32,* 190–198.

DuPaul, G. J., Rapport, M. D., & Perriello, L. M. (1991). Teacher ratings of academic skills: The development of the Academic Performance Rating Scale. *School Psychology Review, 20,* 284–300.

DuPaul, G. J., & Stoner, G. (1994). *ADHD in the schools: Assessment and intervention strategies.* New York: Guilford Press.

Ehrhardt, K. E., Barnett, D. W., Lentz, F. E., Stollar, S. A., & Reifin, L. H. (1996). Innovative methodology in ecological consultation: Use of scripts to promote treatment acceptability and integrity. *School Psychology Quarterly, 11,* 149–168.

Elliott, S. N. (1988). Acceptability of behavioral treatments: Review of variables that influence treatment selection. *Professional Psychology Research and Practice, 19,* 68–80.

Epstein, J. L. (1991). Effects on student achievement of teacher practices and parent involvement. In S. Silvern (Ed.), *Literacy through family, community, and school interaction.* Greenwich, CT: JAI.

Fantuzzo, J. W., Davis, G. Y., & Ginsberg, M. D. (1995). Effects of parent involvement in isolation or in combination with peer tutoring on student self-concept and mathematics achievement. *Journal of Educational Psychology, 87,* 272–281.

Firestone, P., & Witt, J. E. (1982). Characteristics of families completing and prematurely discontinuing a behavioral parent-training program. *Journal of Pediatric Psychology, 7,* 209–222.

Forehand, R., & Scarboro, M. E. (1975). An analysis of children's oppositional behavior. *Journal of Abnormal Child Psychology, 3,* 27–31.

Forehand, R. L., & McMahon, R. J. (1981). *Helping the noncompliant child: A clinician's guide to parent training.* New York: Guilford Press.

Fowler, M. (1992). *CH.A.D.D. educators manual.* Fairfax, VA: CASET.

Foyle, H. C. (1984). The effects of preparation and practice homework on student achievement in tenth-grade American history. *Dissertation Abstracts International, 45,* 2474A.

Frankel, F., Myatt, R., Cantwell, D. P., & Feinberg, D. T. (1997). Parent-assisted transfer of children's social skills training: Effects on children with and without attention deficit hyperactivity disorder. *Journal of the American Academy of Child and Adolescent Psychiatry, 36,* 1056–1064.

Gadow, K. (1997). *Manual for the ADHD Symptom Checklist–4.* Stony Brook, NY: Checkmate Plus.

Garbarino, J., & Abramowitz, R. H. (1992). *Children and families in the social environment.* New York: de Gruyter Press.

Gickling, E., & Thompson, V. P. (1985). A personal view of curriculum-based assessment. *Exceptional Children, 52,* 205–218.

Gresham, F. M. (1989). Assessment of treatment integrity in school consultation and prereferral intervention. *School Psychology Review, 18,* 37–50.

Habboushe, D. F., Daniel, S., Karustis, J. L., Leff, S. S., Costigan, T. E., Goldstein, S. G., Eiraldi, R. B., & Power, T. J. (in press). A family–school homework intervention program for children with attention-deficit/hyperactivity disorder. *Cognitive and Behavioral Practice.*

Ho, B. S. (1997). The school psychologist's role based on an ecological approach to family–school–community collaborations. *California School Psychologist, 11,* 31–38.

Hollingshead, A. B. (1975). *Four-Factor Index of Social Status.* New Haven, CT: Yale University Department of Sociology.

Jayanthi, M., Sawyer, V., Nelson, J. S., Bursuck, W. D., & Epstein, M. H. (1995). Recommendations for homework-communication problems from parents, classroom teachers, and special education teachers. *Remedial and Special Education, 16,* 212–225.

Joost, J. C., Chessare, J. B., Schaeufele, J., Link, D., & Weaver, M. T. (1989). Compliance with a prescription for psychotherapeutic counseling in childhood. *Journal of Developmental and Behavioral Pediatrics, 10,* 98–102.

Kahle, A. L., & Kelley, M. L. (1994). Children's homework problems: A comparison of goal setting and parent training. *Behavior Therapy, 25,* 275–290.

Karustis, J. L., Habboushe, D. F., & Power, T. J. (1997). Facts and misconceptions about ADHD: A guide for psychologists. *Pennsylvania Psychologist Quarterly, 57,* 18–19, 28.

Karustis, J. L., Power, T. J., Rescorla, L. A., Eiraldi, R. B., & Gallagher, P. R. (1998). *The contribution of internalizing symptoms to functional impairment in children with attention-deficit/hyperactivity disorder.* Manuscript submitted for publication.

Kaufman, A. S., & Kaufman, N. L. (1985). *Kaufman Tests of Educational Achievement (K-TEA)–Brief Form.* Circle Pines, MN: American Guidance Service.

Kaufman, A. S., & Kaufman, N. L. (1990). *Kaufman Brief Intelligence Test (K-BIT).* Circle Pines, MN: American Guidance Service.

Kay, P. J., Fitzgerald, M., Paradee, C., & Mellencamp, A. (1994). Making homework work at home: The parent's perspective. *Journal of Learning Disabilities, 27,* 550–561.

Kazdin, A. (1997). Parent management training: Evidence, outcomes, and issues. *Journal of the American Academy of Child and Adolescent Psychiatry, 36,* 1349–1356.

Kazdin, A. E. (1980). Acceptability of alternative treatments for deviant child behavior. *Journal of Applied Behavior Analysis, 13,* 259–273.

Kazdin, A. E., Siegel, T. C., & Bass, D. (1992). Cognitive problem-solving skills training and parent management training in the treatment of antisocial behavior in children. *Journal of Consulting and Clinical Psychology, 60,* 733–747.

Keith, T. Z., & Benson, M. J. (1992). Effects of manipulable influences on high school grades across five ethnic groups. *Journal of Educational Research, 86,* 85–93.

Keith, T. Z., & DeGraff, M. (1997). Homework. In G. G. Bear, K. M. Minke, & A. Thomas (Eds.), *Childrens needs: II. Development, problems, and alternatives.* Bethesda, MD: National Association of School Psychologists.

Keith, T. Z., Keith, P. B., Troutman, G. C., Bickley, P., Trivette, P. S., & Singh, K. (1993). Does parental involvement affect eighth grade student achievement? Structural analysis of national data. *School Psychology Review, 22,* 474–496.

Kelley, M. L. (1990). *School–home notes: Promoting children's classroom success.* New York: Guilford Press.

Kelley, M. L., Heffer, R. W., Gresham, F. M., & Elliott, S. N. (1989). Development of a modified Treatment Evaluation Inventory. *Journal of Psychopathology and Behavioral Assessment, 11*(3), 235–247.

Klein, R. G., & Abikoff, H. (1997). Behavior therapy and methylphenidate in the treatment of children with ADHD. *Journal of Attention Disorders, 2,* 89–114.

Lahey, B. B., Applegate, B., McBurnett, K., Biederman, J., Greenhill, L., Hynd, G. W., Barkley, R. A., Newcorn, J., Jensen, P., Richters, J., Garfinkel, B., Kerdyk, L., Frick, P. J., Ollendick, T., Perez, D., Hart, E. L., Waldman, I., & Shaffer, D. (1994). *DSM-IV* field trial for attention-deficit hyperactivity disorder in children and adolescents. *American Journal of Psychiatry, 151,* 1673–1685.

Landrum, T. J., Al-Mateen, C. S., Ellis, C. R., Singh, N. N., & Ricketts, R. W. (1993). Educational and classroom management. In L. F. Koziol, C. E. Stout, & D. H. Ruben (Eds.), *Handbook of childhood impulse disorders and ADHD: Theory and practice.* Springfield, IL: Thomas.

Lee, J. F., & Pruitt, K. W. (1979). Homework assignments: Classroom games or teaching tools? *Clearinghouse, 53,* 31–35.

Liu, C., Robin, A. L., Brenner, S., & Eastman, J. (1991). Social acceptability of methylphenidate and behavior modification for the treatment of attention deficit hyperactivity disorder. *Pediatrics, 88,* 560–565.

Lordeman, A. M., & Winett, R. A. (1980). The effects of written feedback to parents and a call-service on student homework submission. *Education and Treatment of Children, 3,* 33–44.

Manz, P. H., Power, T. J., Ginsburg-Block, M., & Dowrick, P. W. (2000). *Community partners: Improving the effectiveness of urban schools and empowering low-income, ethnically diverse community residents.* Manuscript submitted for publication.

McCarney, S. B. (1996). *Manual for the Attention Deficit Disorders Evaluation Scale (ADDES): School and home version rating forms.* Columbia, MO: Hawthorne Educational Systems.

McConnaughy, E. A., DiClemente, C. C., Prochaska, J. O., & Velicer, W. F. (1989). Stages of change in psychotherapy: A follow-up report. *Psychotherapy, 26,* 494–503.

McMahon, R. J., Forehand, R., & Greist, D. L. (1981). Effects of knowledge of social learning principles on enhancing treatment outcome and generalization in a parent training program. *Journal of Consulting and Clinical Psychology, 49,* 526–532.

McMiller, W. P., & Weisz, J. R. (1996). Help-seeking preceding mental health clinic intake among African-American, Latino, and Caucasian youths. *Journal of the American Academy of Child and Adolescent Psychiatry, 35,* 1086–1094.

Mercugliano, M., Power, T. J., & Blum, N. J. (1999). *The clinician's practical guide to attention-deficit/hyperactivity disorder.* Baltimore: Brookes.

Miller, D. L., & Kelley, M. L. (1991). Interventions for improving homework performance: A critical review. *School Psychology Quarterly, 6,* 174–185.

Miller, D. L., & Kelley, M. L. (1994). The use of goal setting and contingency contracting for improving children's homework performance. *Journal of Applied Behavior Analysis, 27,* 73–84.

Moncher, F. J., & Prinz, R. J. (1991). Treatment fidelity in outcome studies. *Clinical Psychology Review, 11,* 247–266.

Moore, L. A., Waguespack, A. M., Wickstrom, K. F., Witt, J. C., & Gaydos, G. R. (1994). Mystery motivator: An effective and time efficient intervention. *School Psychology Review, 23,* 106–118.

Naglieri, J. A., LeBuffe, P. A., & Pfeiffer, S. I. (1994). *Manual for the Devereux Scales of Mental Disorders.* San Antonio, TX: Psychological Corporation.

Nastasi, B. K., Varjas, K., Bernstein, R., & Pluymert, K. (1998). Mental health programming and the role of school psychologists. *School Psychology Review, 27,* 217–232.

Northup, J., Broussard, C., Jones, K., George, T., Vallmer, T., & Herring, M. (1995). The differential effects of teacher and peer attention on the disruptive classroom behavior of three children diagnosed with attention deficit hyperactivity disorder. *Journal of Applied Behavior Analysis, 28,* 277–282.

Olympia, D., Jenson, W. R., Clark, E., & Sheridan, S. (1992). Training parents to facilitate homework completion: A model for home–school collaboration. In S. L. Christenson & J. C. Conoley (Eds.), *Home–school collaboration: Enhancing children's academic and social competence.* Silver Spring, MD: National Association of School Psychologists.

Olympia, D. E., Jenson, W. R., & Hepworth-Neville, M. (1996). *Sanity savers for parents: Tips for tackling homework.* Longmont, CO: SoprisWest.

Olympia, D. E., Sheridan, S. M., & Jenson, W. R. (1994). Homework: A natural means of home–school collaboration. *School Psychology Quarterly, 9,* 60–80.

Olympia, D. E., Sheridan, S. M., Jenson, W. R., & Andrews, D. (1994). Using student-managed interventions to increase homework completion and accuracy. *Journal of Applied Behavior Analysis, 27,* 85–99.

Paschal, R. A., Weinstein, T., & Walberg, H. J. (1984). The effects of homework on learning: A quantitative analysis. *Journal of Educational Research, 78,* 97–104.

Pelham, W. E., Carlson, C., Sams, S. E., Vallano, G., Dixon, M. J., & Hoza, B. (1993). Separate and combined effects of methylphenidate and behavior modification on boys with attention deficit-hyperactivity disorder in the classroom. *Journal of Consulting and Clinical Psychology, 61,* 506–515.

Pfiffner, L. J., & Barkley, R. A. (1998). Treatment of ADHD in school settings. In R. A. Barkley, *Attention-deficit hyperactivity disorder: A handbook for diagnosis and treatment* (2nd ed.). New York: Guilford Press.

Pfiffner, L. J., & O'Leary, S. G. (1993). School-based psychological treatments. In J. L. Matson (Ed.), *Handbook of hyperactivity in children.* Boston: Allyn & Bacon.

Piper, W. E., & Perrault, E. L. (1989). Pretherapy preparation for group members. *International Journal of Group Psychotherapy, 9,* 17–34.

Pisterman, S., McGrath, P., Firestone, P., Goodman, J. T., Webster, I., & Mallory, R. (1989). Outcome of parent-mediated treatment of preschoolers with attention deficit disorder with hyperactivity. *Journal of Consulting and Clinical Psychology, 57,* 628–635.

Power, T. J., Andrews, T. J., Eiraldi, R. B., Doherty, B. J., Ikeda, M. J., DuPaul, G. J., & Landau, S. (1998). Evaluating attention deficit hyperactivity disorder using multiple informants: The incremental utility of combining teacher with parent reports. *Psychological Assessment, 10,* 250–260.

Power, T. J., Atkins, M., Osborne, M., & Blum, N. (1994). The school psychologist as manager of programming for ADHD. *School Psychology Review, 23,* 279–291.

Power, T. J., Dowrick, P. W., Ginsburg-Block, M., & Manz, P. H. (2000). *Building the capacity of urban schools to improve literacy skills: Community-assisted tutoring.* Manuscript submitted for publication.

Power, T. J., & DuPaul, G. J. (1996). Attention-deficit hyperactivity disorder: The reemergence of subtypes. *School Psychology Review, 25,* 284–296.

Power, T. J., Eiraldi, R. B., Mercugliano, M., & Blum, N. J. (1998). Using interviews and rating scales to collect behavioral data. In M. Mercugliano, T. J. Power, & N. J. Blum, *The clinician's practical guide to attention-deficit/hyperactivity disorder.* Baltimore: Brookes.

Power, T. J., Hess, L., & Bennett, D. (1995). The acceptability of interventions for ADHD among elementary and middle school teachers. *Journal of Developmental and Behavioral Pediatrics, 16,* 238–243.

Power, T. J., Karustis, J. L., Mercugliano, M., & Blum, N. J. (1999). Psychoeducational assessment for children with attention-deficit/hyperactivity disorder. In M. Mercugliano, T. J., Power, & N. J. Blum, *The clinician's practical guide to attention-deficit/hyperactivity disorder.* Baltimore: Brookes.

Prochaska, J. O., & DiClemente, C. C. (1992). *Stages of change in the modification of problem behaviors.* Newbury Park, CA: Sage.

Prochaska, J. O., DiClemente, C. C., & Norcross, J. C. (1992). In search of how people change: Applications to addictive behaviors. *American Psychologist, 47,* 1102–1114.

Prochaska, J. O., Velicer, W. F., Rossi, J. S., Goldstein, M. G., Marcus, B. H., Rakowski, W., Fiore, C., Harlow, L. L., Redding, C. A., Rosenbloom, D., & Rossi, S. R. (1994). Stages of change and decisional balance for 12 problem behaviors. *Health Psychology, 13,* 39–46.

Psychological Corporation. (1992). *Wechsler Individual Achievement Test Screener.* San Antonio, TX: Author.

Psychological Corporation (1999). *Wechsler Abbreviated Scale of Intelligence (WASI).* San Antonio, TX: Author.

Pumariega, A. J. (1996). Culturally competent outcome evaluation in systems of care for children's mental health. *Journal of Child and Family Studies, 5,* 389–397.

Rapport, M. D., Stoner, G., DuPaul, G. J., Kelley, K. L., Tucker, S. B., & Schoeler, T. (1988). Attention deficit disorder and methylphenidate: A multilevel analysis of dose–response effects on children's impulsivity across settings. *Journal of the American Academy of Child and Adolescent Psychiatry, 27,* 60–69.

Reich, W., Leacock, N., & Shanfeld, K. (1995). *Diagnostic Interview for Children and Adolescents: DSM-IV Revision (Parent Form).* St. Louis, MO: Washington University.

Reid, R. (1995). Assessment of ADHD with culturally different groups: The use of behavior rating scales for identifying students with ADHD. *School Psychology Review, 24,* 537–560.

Reimers, T. M., Wacker, D. P., Cooper, L. J., & DeRaad, A. O. (1992). Acceptability of behavioral treatments for children: Analog and naturalistic evaluation by parents. *School Psychology Review, 21,* 628–643.

Reimers, T. M., Wacker, D. P., & Koeppl, G. (1987). Acceptability of behavioral interventions: A review of the literature. *School Psychology Review, 16*(2), 212–227.

Reynolds, C. R., & Kamphaus, R. W. (1992). *Manual for the Behavior Assessment System for Children.* Circle Pines, MN: American Guidance Service.

Rhoades, M. M., & Kratochwill, T. R. (1998). Parent training and consultation: An analysis of a homework intervention program. *School Psychology Quarterly, 13,* 241–264.

Richters, J. E., Arnold, L. E., Jensen, P. S., & Abikoff, H. (1995). NIMH collaborative multisite multimodal treatment study of children with ADHD: I. Background and rationale. *Journal of the American Academy of Child and Adolescent Psychiatry, 34,* 987–1000.

Robin, A. L. (1998). Training families with ADHD adolescents. In R. A. Barkley, *Attention-deficit hyperactivity disorder: A handbook for diagnosis and treatment* (2nd ed.). New York: Guilford Press.

Robin, A. L., & Foster, S. L. (1989). *Negotiating parent–adolescent conflict: A behavioral–family systems approach.* New York: Guilford Press.

Schoenholtz-Read, J. (1994). Selection of group intervention. In H. S. Bernard & K. R. MacKenzie (Eds.), *Basics of group psychotherapy*. New York: Guilford Press.

Schwartz, I. S., & Baer, D. M. (1991). Social validity assessments: Is current practice state of the art? *Journal of Applied Behavior Analysis, 24*, 189–204.

Shapiro, E. S. (1996). *Academic skills problems: Direct assessment and intervention* (2nd ed.). New York: Guilford Press.

Shapiro, E. S., DuPaul, G. J., Bradley, K. L., & Bailey, L. T. (1996). A school-based consultation program for service delivery to middle school students with attention-deficit/hyperactivity disorder. *Journal of Emotional and Behavioral Disorders, 4*, 73–81.

Sheridan, S. M., Kratochwill, T. R., & Bergan, J. R. (1996). *Conjoint Behavioral Consultation: A procedural manual*. New York: Plenum Press.

Shriver, M. D., & Allen, K. D. (1996). The time-out grid: A guide to effective discipline. *School Psychology Quarterly, 11*, 67–74.

Szatmari, P., Offord, D. R., & Boyle, M. H. (1989). Ontario Child Health Study: Prevalence of attention deficit disorder with hyperactivity. *Journal of Child Psychology and Psychiatry, 30*, 219–230.

Ullman, R. K., Sleator, E. K., Sprague, R. K., & MetriTech Staff (1996). *Manual for the Comprehensive Teacher's Rating Scale: Parent Form (ACTeRS)*. Champaign, IL: MetriTech.

Vance, H. B. (Ed.). (1997). *Psychological assessment of children: Best practices for school and clinical settings* (2nd ed.). New York: Wiley.

Vinogradov, S., & Yalom, I. D. (1989). *A concise guide to group psychotherapy*. Washington, DC: American Psychiatric Press.

Wahler, R. G., & Dumas, J. E. (1989). Attentional problems in dysfunctional mother–child interactions: An interbehavioral model. *American Psychologist, 105*, 116–130.

Webster-Stratton, C., & Hammond, M. (1997). Treating children with early-onset conduct problems: A comparison of child and parent interventions. *Journal of Consulting and Clinical Psychology, 65*, 93–109.

Wechsler, D. (1991). *The Wechsler Intelligence Scale for Children–Third Edition*. New York: Psychological Cooperation.

Weiner, R. K., Sheridan, S. M., & Jenson, W. R. (1998). The effects of conjoint behavioral consultation and a structured homework program on math completion and accuracy in junior high school students. *School Psychology Quarterly, 13*, 281–309.

Weiss, G., & Hechtman, L. T. (1993). *Hyperactive children grown up* (2nd ed): *ADHD in children, adolescents, and adults*. New York: Guilford Press.

Witt, J. C., & Elliott, S. N. (1985). Acceptability of classroom intervention strategies. In T. R. Kratochwill (Ed.), *Advances in school psychology* (Vol. 4). Hillsdale, NJ: Erlbaum.

Yalom, I. D. (1975). *The theory and practice of group psychotherapy* (2nd ed.). New York: Basic Books.

Zentall, S. (1993). Research on the educational implications of attention deficit disorder. *Exceptional Children, 60*, 143–153.

Zentall, S. S., & Dwyer, A. M. (1988). Color effects on the impulsivity and activity of hyperactive children. *Journal of School Psychology, 27*, 165–174.

Index

G

H